Terpenes for Well-Being

A Comprehensive Guide to Botanical Aromas for Emotional and Physical Self-Care

Andrew Freedman

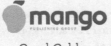

Coral Gables

For permission requests, please contact the publisher at:

Mango Publishing Group
2850 Douglas Road, 2nd Floor
Coral Gables, FL 33134 USA
info@mango.bz

For special orders, quantity sales, course adoptions and corporate sales, please email the publisher at sales@mango.bz. For trade and wholesale sales, please contact Ingram Publisher Services at customer.service@ ingramcontent.com or +1.800.509.4887.

Terpenes for Well-Being: A Comprehensive Guide to Botanical Aromas for Emotional and Physical Self-Care

ISBN: (p) 978-1-64250-552-8 (e) 978-1-64250-553-5
BISAC: HEA029000, HEALTH & FITNESS / Aromatherapy
LCCN: 2021931913

Praise for *Terpenes for Well-Being*

"Terpenes are the hidden secret behind cannabis and healing. Without the essential aromatics, there would be no differences between cultivars and the way cannabis affects our bodies. I'm proud to give a tip of my hat to Andrew for his research and careful recommendations in the olfactory world of sensory memories."

—**Warren Bobrow,** author of *The Cocktail Compendium* and *Cannabis Cocktails, Mocktails & Tonics,* CEO of Klaus Apothicaire, cannabis alchemist, and master mixologist

"*Terpenes for Well-Being* is a great source of knowledge for food and beverage professionals, as well as enthusiasts seeking cannabis and botanical-related holistic wellness information. In this primer, noted mixologist and cannabis industry expert Andrew Freedman demystifies terpenes, by shining a spotlight on the many flavors, effects, and potential benefits of terpenes, and explores how to utilize your senses of smell, taste, and beyond. Whether you are new to handling or consuming cannabis, have an interest in aromatherapy, or want to expand your culinary repertoire to include the basics of natural plant terpenes, you'll enjoy this book!"

—**Jacqui Pressinger,** director of strategic partnerships for the American Culinary Federation

"*Terpenes for Well-Being* is a delightful and informative guide for those of us who want to enjoy our sense of taste and smell. From wellness applications to encouragement of mental health practices and showing us an understanding what makes humans tick, Andrew Freedman offers a wild adventure for the senses rarely explored in books."

—**Dean Barker**, The Food Network

"*Terpenes for Well-Being* by Andrew Freedman is the newest book that you need to add to your cannabis education book collection. Andrew uncovers cannabis, terpenes, infused food, and aromatherapy for self-care in an easily relatable and obtainable fashion. Andrew Freedman's book is a needed addition to any cannabis education or aromatherapy collection.

—**Respect My Region**, online lifestyle and music platform

Terpenes for Well-Being

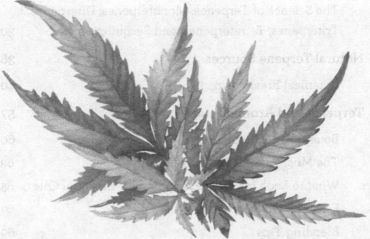

Table of Contents

Preface

Until you dive down the right rabbit hole, many subjects remain shrouded in mystery. It's easy to get caught up in using words without taking the time to fully understand them.

I have a lot of conversations about "terps," a widely referenced term for the aroma of cannabis. But what are "terps," and how do we create a better understanding of them? When I say terps, I am of course using the shorthand term for terpenes.

Our senses are bombarded daily, and none more so than our sense of smell. Like it or not, you will smell whatever is around you. But what are smells? Where do they come from, and how can we understand them better?

—Andrew Freedman

Introduction

We are always surrounded by smells. No matter where we go, memories are evoked by fragrances wafting in the air. But what are these aromas we so lovingly odor...I mean *adore*? Where do they come from, and how do they get there? The simple answer is terpenes! A longer answer to those questions, however, is found in the pages of this book.

Throughout the book, we will learn to identify natural terpene sources and how to utilize them in everyday life for self-care and wellness. By the end of this book, you will (hopefully) be able to identify many different aromas and the terpene building blocks of which they are made by their smell, use terpenes and essential oils in lotions, baths, and aromatherapy, learn some incredible original recipes utilizing natural terpene sources, and become intimately familiar with the process of cooking with cannabis.

Our tongues can only taste five things: sour, sweet, salty, bitter, and umami. But we can smell millions of combinations that have the power to transport us back to particular moments of our lives, filling us with emotion. Why does smell have such a strong connection to emotion?

It seems so simple to stop and smell the roses, doesn't it? It is the act of merely taking a moment to enjoy one of our physical senses, perhaps the one that is most complex, yet taken for granted—smell. This is the foundation of this book:

the willingness to take the time to stop, think, and enjoy each smell for the simple yet complex combination that it is.

I have been in the cannabis trade for over a decade. Cannabis cultivators often engage in informal rivalry as to whose flowers smell the best (as opposed to just the most strongly, i.e., "skunk weed"). I thought there must be a way to prove that one cannabis grower's bud does smell better than another's. I became instantly fascinated with the world of wine and blind tasting and moved to a vineyard to become a winemaker's apprentice. It was there my eyes were opened to the deep and intense world of flavor and smell waiting to be explored. I became so excited about earning accreditation while developing my palate that I became a Canadian Wine Scholar and earned a Level Three certification in wine from the Wine & Spirit Education Trust (WSET). While working in the wine trade and starting a YouTube channel, I was able to taste thousands of wines and cannabis strains. My love and exploration of new and unique smells and flavors led me to want to explore further and, inevitably, to write a book.

Many of us think of aroma as a linear concept, a characteristic made up of easy to identify elements. We've all heard people say things like, "This smells like cookies," or "that smells like a bouquet of flowers," but what really is the source of that aroma? We will dissect what really creates each combination of scents; as a result, you will not only become more aware of the pieces that make up specific aromas, but you'll learn about the building blocks of how the smell of chocolate chip cookies came to be.

Although terpenes are nothing new—research chemist Otto Wallach won a Nobel Prize back in 1910 for his revolutionary work on terpenes—the conversation around them is. The rapid legalization of cannabis at a nearly global level is the largest driving factor for the increased interest in terpenes. Terpenes have been utilized in aromatherapy for the last one hundred years, evoking effects of relaxation, euphoria, relief from depression, and so much more. But they have not been thought about deeply as single source molecules which create complex and effervescent aromas.

When I was growing up, my mom loved teaching me about aromatherapy. I am truly amazed at how much of it has stuck with me through my life. From lemon-scented anxiety rollers to essential oil diffusers, little did I know I was being led down a path of natural self-care and wellness.

This book is a collection of all the best-smelling and most delicious things I could think of. It's an amazing bonus that most of them also have incredible and powerful healing properties.

Together, we will smell deeper than you may have ever considered possible. We will peel back the layers that create aromas and learn to identify the source terpene molecules and their building blocks. We will also look at how these terpenes and essential oils can be derived from naturally originating materials and how they have shaped our perceptions of smell.

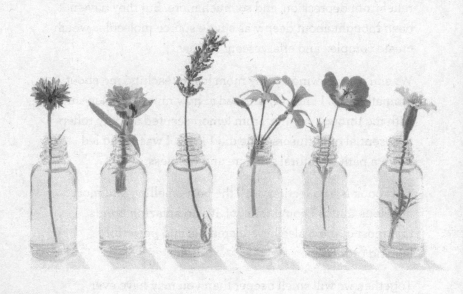

Blueberry, marigold, in bloom lavender, geranium, pelargonium, and yellow carnation essential oils.

What Are Terpenes?

You have been experiencing terpenes your entire life, even if this is the first time you've heard the word. Simply put, terpenes are what make oranges smell like citrus and pine trees smell like pine, and they are also responsible for the calming effects of lavender. Terpenes are the chemicals that make things have a scent.

Terpenes are single-molecule building blocks of essential oils produced by most plants. Fruit, leaves, roots, flowers, and even some animals produce terpenes! Terpenes are volatile aromatic compounds that easily react with oxygen, evaporating and becoming aerosols.

Strong smelling plants and flowers evolved their aromas, essential oils, and terpene compounds through untold generations for adaptive purposes—mainly to repel predators and attract pollinators in the wild. Some terpenes play a protective role, aiding the plant in recovery from damage or acting as part of the plant's immune system to keep away infection. There are many elements that influence the development of terpenes, but a lemon will always smell like a lemon.

Each terpene has its own distinct scent, which plays a major role in defining flavor and aroma. But much in the same way that you can't taste eggs in a cake, all terpenes, as well as other aromatic compounds, come together to create a unique and special symphony of smell.

There are over 20,000 different terpenes in existence! The cannabis plant, for example, has over a hundred terpenes in its various varietals. We can also credit terpenes (as well as flavonoids) for the taste and aroma of our favorite wine or beer! What did you think those hops were *really* doing?

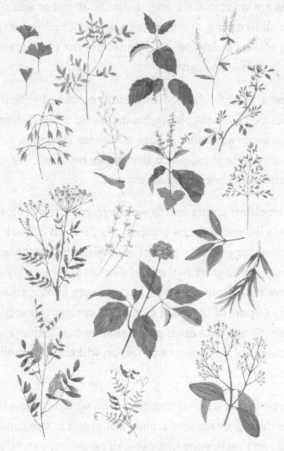

Culinary and medicinal herbs.

How Terpenes Work

Terpenes are bioactive compounds, which means they affect the body. The effect of a terpene will vary based on its concentration and other characteristics and the body of the person who uses it. Our individual biology is unique, and we must understand that we are not all affected in the same way.

Because terpenes form vibrant smells, they are used as the building blocks for essential oils, which are integral parts of many alternative therapies like aromatherapy. Inhaling the scents from plants and essential oils may affect and alter a person's mood or stress levels.

Terpenes also play a major role in the intoxicating effects of cannabis. Terpenes affect and enhance cannabis intoxication through what has been coined the "entourage effect." The entourage effect implies that terpenes enhance and alter the effects of cannabinoids when inhaled. There is lots of research that backs up these claims.

There is also plenty of medical research that has been done on isolated terpenes; some may even make their way into medical use. Terpenes have been shown to have many beneficial effects on the body and could serve as alternative medicines and therapies. We will dive further into this later in the book.

Using Terpenes Safely

Any essential oil has the potential to cause a skin reaction when applied topically. If you are worried about a possible reaction, test a small amount of any terpene or essential oil on the inside of your elbow in a diluted form before using it on any larger areas.

Avoid using old or oxidized terpenes or essential oils as these can cause dermal sensitization. This is a type of allergic reaction that may not be noticeable after one use but, at times, essential oils can cause severe adverse effects if used repeatedly.

Some citrus essential oils are phototoxic and can cause painful skin reactions if you use them on your skin and then go outside in the sun.

Follow these safety precautions for best results when using terpenes and essential oils:

◆ Don't apply undiluted essential oils or terpenes to your skin.

◆ Keep oils and terpenes away from your eyes.

◆ Store oils and terpenes safely out of reach of children or other vulnerable individuals.

◆ When vaporizing your oils or terpenes for aromatherapy, make sure the area is well ventilated.

◆ If you are pregnant, breastfeeding, or taking prescription medications, it is always best to consult with your doctor.

Types of Terpenes

As previously mentioned, thousands of terpenes have been discovered, but only a fraction have been explored. Terpenes are the fragrant oils responsible for giving a multitude of plants their unique smell and taste. There is an extremely diverse range of aromas found in terpenes. They can present with woody, earthy, floral, fruity, citrusy, spicy, or sweet aromas. Interestingly, there are many terpenes that are unique to cannabis.

We all have individual preferences for smells and taste so knowing the profile of different terpenes can be very beneficial in choosing aromatherapy or cannabis products. Understanding terpenes can help you to best select or even create the scent and flavor profile you desire.

Different terpenes are often associated with different naturopathic remedies, and some theorize that they play an important role in the effects of cannabis intoxication and medication. This theory is discussed later in the book in the section on the entourage effect.

Let's discuss some of the most popular terpenes.

Limonene

Limonene is easily the most recognizable terpene, and you can probably guess what it tastes like just from the name: lemons! But not just lemons, limonene is partly responsible for the familiar smells of all citrus fruits. High concentrations of limonene can be found in lemons, limes, grapefruits, and orange rinds. This scent is often associated with an uplifted and energized feeling. It is also a "clean" aroma, which is one of the reasons why it is one of the leading terpenes used to add scent to cleaning products.

Studies show that limonene has several positive therapeutic properties; it is anti-inflammatory, antioxidant, antiviral, and antidiabetic, among its useful properties.

Limonene seems to modulate the way certain immune cells behave, which may protect the body from a range of disorders. Limonene can be taken as a supplement all on its own for its known positive effects.

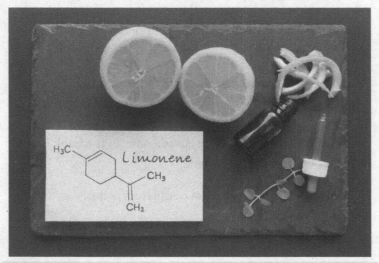

Structural chemical formula of limonene with fresh citrus—limonene is the major component in the oil of citrus peels.

Pinene

Pinene may be the most abundant terpene, at least around me in the Rocky Mountains! You may be able to guess pinene's source by its name: pine trees! The alluring smell of the forest is made up of a plethora of aerosol terpenes. There are two forms of pinene, alpha-pinene and beta-pinene, written as α-pinene and β-pinene. Pinene provides the bright fresh scent of many plants including pine needles, basil, and rosemary. Pinene also has some reported therapeutic effects.

In Japan, *shirin-yoku* is a therapy that includes taking leisurely walks through the forest, enjoying its scent and soaking up the atmosphere. *Shirin-yoku* is translated as "forest bathing." Inhaling the pinene aerosols released by the trees is believed to have restorative effects on a person's physical and metaphysical well-being, as well as preventing some illnesses.

Studies show that the amount of aerosol pinene in the air of a healthy forest is enough to be therapeutic. Pinene works as a bronchodilator, allowing more air into your lungs. It is also an anti-inflammatory and may help the body resist some types of infectious germs when inhaled.

Pine trees give a sense of floating terpenes.

Linalool

Linalool is responsible for the smell of lavender plants and gives the lavender flower its rich and alluring scent. Linalool is one of the most important compounds in aromatherapy and causes the calming effect many people experience when smelling lavender or its essential oils. (This explains why bubble bath and bath salts are often scented with linalool.)

Linalool has a wide range of properties that can affect the body in many ways. It has been shown that linalool has anti-inflammatory, antimicrobial, neuroprotective, antidepressant, and antianxiety properties.

Linalool clearly has an effect on the human body, but there has not yet been enough medical research on it to definitively say how it can be used to benefit your health. Linalool is classified as a monoterpene.

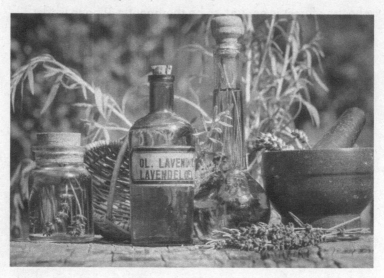

Lavender flowers and lavender essential oil.

Myrcene

Myrcene is a monoterpene commonly found in mangoes and the herbs hops, lemon grass, and thyme. Myrcene is also the most commonly found terpene in cannabis plants!

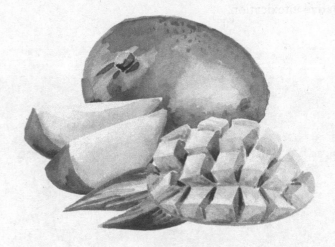

Mango and mango cubes.

Myrcene is a powerful antioxidant. Studies on mice have shown it may help protect the brain from oxidative damage following a stroke. Another study found a similar protective effect on the heart tissue of mice. Researchers noted that myrcene may be an effective therapy after suffering a stroke. (These studies used very high doses of myrcene, the use of which should only be undertaken if prescribed by your own physician.)

Other studies have shown that myrcene appears to have anti-inflammatory properties that are useful when dealing with osteoarthritis.

When inhaled, myrcene creates a more permeable layer in the blood-brain barrier in humans. This may be why the cannabis strains that are highest in myrcene give us the most sedative intoxication.

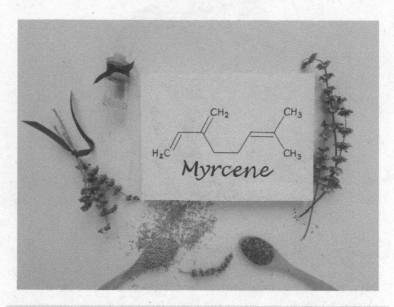

The structural chemical formula of the myrcene molecule, surrounded by basil and rosemary.

Beta-Caryophyllene

Beta-caryophyllene exists in many herbs and vegetables, such as clove and black pepper. It adds the spicy note that is characteristic when tasting that first crack of pepper.

Similar to other terpenes, beta-caryophyllene may have some anti-inflammatory properties and may help reduce pain levels in some people.

Studies have shown that beta-caryophyllene can reduce pain and nerve pain. Research noted that its anti-inflammatory and analgesic effect might be useful for treating long-term chronic pain because the research subjects showed no sign of developing a tolerance to beta-caryophyllene's useful effects.

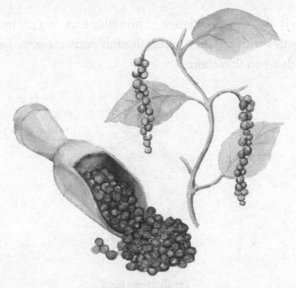

Dried black pepper and black pepper.

Humulene

Humulene was discovered while researching the terpenes found in cannabis plants. While searching for a relative of this terpene, it was discovered that the common hops plant, (with the scientific name *Humulus lupulus*), shared a similar biochemical profile with cannabis. Hence the terpene found in both was named humulene, or the "hoppy" terpene. Other plants like clove and ginger also contain humulene.

One study showed that humulene may have the potential to prevent allergic reactions and asthma. In research on animals, humulene has been shown to reduce inflammation in the airways. This means it could potentially be helpful as a natural asthma treatment.

There is also other evidence of humulene having protective properties with regard to cells, though more research needs to be done on this claim.

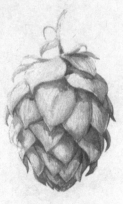

Fresh green hop.

Menthol

Menthol is a terpene found in its highest concentrations in peppermint and spearmint. Menthol is cooling and minty and so is often added to items in need of flavoring. Menthol is one of the most popular terpenes in the world.

Menthol may also be the most medically researched of all terpenes. A lot of studies have been done on its effects on human health. Mint has been shown to improve irritable bowel syndrome and relieve indigestion. Menthol is a fantastic decongestant often utilized for symptoms of the flu or the common cold. Menthol appears in many over-the-counter health products and is used in a large number of essential oil blends.

The majority of medical studies on menthol have focused on its ability to improve lung function. The most commonly known menthol-rich and commercially available topical salve is Vicks VapoRub. Consisting of 2.6 percent menthol, this is a common ointment for relieving congestion and easing coughing. It's also known to soothe sore muscles.

Menthol has been found to be antibacterial; it can also inhibit the growth of fungi and can be used to treat some skin conditions. Menthol used externally produces a numbing sensation that can help with itchy bug bites or carpet burn. Be warned, do *not* apply menthol directly to a wound as it may burn. Menthol is also known to relieve joint pain and headaches, reduce acne, and ease asthma.

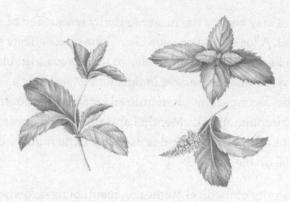

A collection of mint leaves.

All of the terpenes covered above are among the most prominent, widely used, and most researched today. All of them are found in a broad spectrum of plants, and research is ongoing into newly isolated terpenes to determine their particular qualities and medicinal benefits. With so many terpenes being discovered (including over one hundred in the cannabis plant alone), it is best to highlight the most common terpenes.

You will find a combination of many of these terpenes in various proportions in most essential oils. Terpenes can be utilized for many things, from making rubber to manufacturing steroids.

Maple syrup contains over three hundred terpenes, eh!

Other Terpenes

Listed above are the most popular terpenes that one may come across while exploring. As mentioned earlier, there are over 20,000 noted terpenes and many yet to be discovered. Here are some of the other prominent terpenes that we will come across later in the book:

Borneol—Smells like menthol, camphor, and rich earth. It is found in wormwood and cinnamon.

Carene—Smells like earth, pine, and forest and is found in bell pepper, pine, and citrus fruits.

Cedrene—Smells like cedar, amber, sandalwood, and patchouli. It is found in cedar bark.

Citronellol—Smells like florals, sweet citrus, and rose. It is found in roses, geraniums, and lemongrass.

Geraniol—Smells like geranium, rose, citronella, and stone fruits and is found in geraniums, tobacco, and lemons.

Linalool—Smells like sweet flowers and citrus and is found in lavender (as well as many other flowers), mint, and cinnamon.

Nerol—Smells like bitter orange, citrus, and rose. It is found in cumin, lilac, apple, tea tree, and conifers.

Nerolidol—Smells like wood, bark, flowers, and apples; it is found in citronella, ginger, and orange peel.

Ocimene—Smells like flowers, fruit, and herbs and is found in mint, parsley, pepper, basil, mango, and orchids.

Sabinene—Smells like wood, pepper, and spices and found in oak, tea tree oil, black pepper, and carrot seed.

Terpineol—Smells like florals, lilac, lime, cardamom, and clove. It is found in cypress, juniper berries, cardamom, marjoram, and thyme.

The Science of Terpenes: Monoterpenes, Diterpenes, Triterpenes, Tetraterpenes, and Sesquiterpenes

Terpenoids, or terpenes, are an extremely large and diverse group of naturally occurring compounds. Terpenes are mostly found in plants, but some terpenes such as squalene are present in animals. Terpenes are responsible for the fragrance, taste, and sometimes the pigment of a plant.

A terpene can fall into a number of given classes, including mono, sesqui, di, tri, or tetra terpenes, all of which are found in nature. Isoprenes are bonding units, and a terpene is classified into one of these categories by how many isoprenes it contains. Think of isoprenes as the building blocks of terpenes.

Terpenes provide major protective benefits to plant organisms. You are probably already familiar with many commonly found terpene-rich plant sources, like lemon, grapefruit, lime, thyme, cannabis, tea, or sage. Terpenes protect plants by warding off viruses, bacteria, pathogens, and predators. It is extremely interesting how different plants have evolved to use terpenes for common purposes even though the terpenes are present in different amounts and varieties.

Terpenes have a wide range of valuable medicinal characteristics, including antiparasitic effects. Interestingly, the antiparasitic properties of terpenes act in a way similar to the popular malaria drug chloroquine. Monoterpenes specifically are being studied for their antiviral properties. Terpenes have the potential to treat many ailments ranging across the spectrum from the common flu to some cancers.

Terpenes and essential oils have been widely used in traditional medicine for centuries for their noted positive effects. They are also widely used to remedy the side effects of other drugs. Many terpene-rich aromatherapeutic essential oils also help with peripheral anxiety and stress caused by various ailments.

Curcumin is an interesting terpene widely used in folk medicines, one which has powerful antiseptic, anti-inflammatory, antioxidant and digestive properties. Curcumin has become a recent trend in health foods, opening the doors for new research on it.

Here's a summary of various types of terpenes, their sources, medicinal properties, and methods of action, and a few studies showing the importance of terpenes and associated molecular compounds in modern medicine.

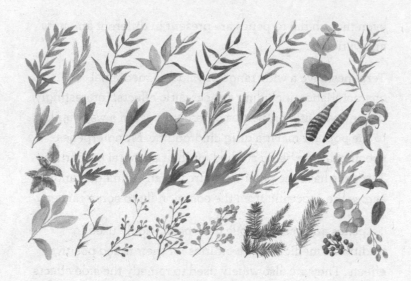

Various plant leaves and branches.

Monoterpenes

The smallest terpenes are monoterpenes. Derived from flowers, fruits, and leaves, they contain the compound $C_{10}H_{16}$, or terpinene, and are considered the key component of essential oils, fragrances and many structural isomers. Monoterpenes are also the most fragrant of all the classes of terpenes. Two examples of the monoterpenes in natural scents are α-pinene, which imparts scent to pine trees, and limonene from citrus plants.

The main purposes of monoterpenes are probably attracting pollinators or repelling other organisms from feeding on host plants. Monoterpenes are isolated from their plant sources by steam distillation at boiling points in the range of 150 to 185 degrees Celsius.

Note: Though terpenes exist in cannabis, levels and kinds differ across its many strains. Terpenes add an incredible dimension to how cannabinoids function in the body, and while they may not all get you "high," their therapeutic effects are likely to have a positive impact on your overall health.

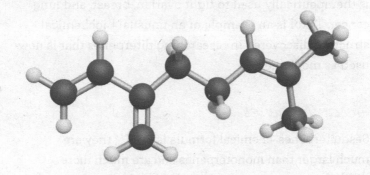

Myrcene
C10H16

bay, cannabis, cardamom, hops, lemon grass, thyme

Structure of myrcene.

Diterpenes

Diterpenes are an interesting naturally occurring terpene group whose members all have the molecular formula $C_{20}H_{32}$. Diterpenes contain biochemicals like vitamin A and hormones that promote plant growth and regulate germination, flowering, and reproductive cycles (sexual to asexual or vice versa). Diterpenes have been shown to have antitumor and anti-inflammatory properties. Diterpenes have attracted increasing attention due to their interesting biological and pharmacological activities. Although thousands of diterpene compounds from terrestrial and marine organisms in nature have been described, only a few of them have so far been proven clinically effective. One effective example of a diterpene used for medicine is taxol. Taxol is a diterpene used to make the anticancer chemotherapy drug Taxotere. Taxol (Taxotere) is therapeutically used to fight ovarian, breast, and lung cancer. Taxol is an example of an unusual biochemical structure discovered in researching diterpenes that is now used as medicine.

Sesquiterpenes

Sesquiterpenes' chemical formula is $C_{15}H_{24}$; they are much larger than monoterpenes and are much more stable in comparison, meaning they don't evaporate and oxidize as quickly. Sesquiterpenes are found in plants, fungi, and insects. In insects, sesquiterpenes act as pheromones. Some sesquiterpene compounds, such as farnesan, are used on insects as natural pesticides. They can also be used by mammals like elephants to mark their territory. Sesquiterpenes seem to play a vital role in plant development and the release of growth hormones and are also involved in plants' ability to sense and adjust to conditions in their environment. The medicinal properties of sesquiterpenes typically come from flowering plants of the Asteraceae family, including daisies, marigolds, and sunflowers. Sesquiterpenes have been used in medicine for their anti-inflammatory, anticancer, and antiviral properties,

Sesquiterpenes are also found to reduce stomach ulcers. These same terpenes are utilized in powerful antimalarial drugs as well.

Triterpenes

Triterpenes are composed of either three or six isoprene units and have a chemical formula of $C_{30}H_{48}$. They include steroids and sterols, and the isoprene squalene is the biological foundation of all triterpenes. Triterpenes are produced by animals, plants, and fungi, and they play a major role as precursors to steroids both in plants and animals.

The medicinal uses of triterpenes are not as well recognized as those of most other types of terpenes, but research on their uses is ongoing. Triterpenes have been studied for anticancer, antioxidant, antiviral, and anti-atherosclerotic properties, i.e., reducing the plaque and fats that clog artery walls.

Other studies indicate a fascinating dual potential for antidiabetic uses of triterpenes, both to reduce glucose levels and to inhibit the human body's response to sweetness in sweet and high calorie foods. Triterpenes have been found to lessen glucose and insulin responses to high carbohydrate meals.

Tetraterpenes

Tetraterpenes, or carotenoids, have a molecular formula of $C_{40}H_{56}$. Although tetraterpenes are not primarily fragrant, they are made of isoprenes, meaning they are technically classified as terpenes. Tetraterpenes are found in many different types of plants, bacteria, and fungi. Tetraterpenes are the primary cause of red, yellow, and orange fat-soluble plant and animal pigments. One of the most important and common tetraterpenes is the well-known beta-carotene, which results in the yellow/orange pigment in carrots. It is important to mammals for producing vitamin A and other important terpenoids related to vision.

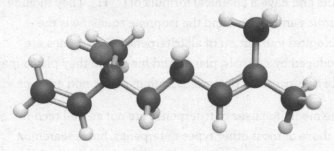

(S)-Linalool
$C_{10}H_{18}O$
basil, cannabis, citrus, coriander, laurel, lavender

Chemical structure of linalool.

A Quick Summary

Terpenes are the aromatic compounds that give plants their distinct smells. Many plants contain varying levels of complex terpenes. Terpenes all play specific roles in a plant's life, such as attracting pollinators, repelling pests, and helping the plant resist disease. Terpenes play a clear role in the health and survival of plants, and they are abundant in many aromatic plants found all over the world. In some cases, smelling specific terpene-rich essential oils, ingesting terpene-rich plants, or spending time near plants with high terpene content may provide health benefits to humans.

Let's find out where we can find some abundant sources of terpenes in our everyday lives and how we can start incorporating them into our everyday lives for self-care and improved well-being.

Natural
Terpene Sources

Terpenes are all around us. We can think of them as the building blocks of smell. If aroma is composed of terpenes, then we can understand that any scent is just a combination of volatile terpenes, alcohols, and esters. This combination forms essential oils, which are some of the most complex and powerful elements in nature. Essential oils are created in nature, by nature, for natural purposes like helping plants survive and thrive while deterring pests and bacteria.

Essential oils are the life force of a plant—a form of concentrated energy that allows a plant to function as it should.

Essential oils aren't actually oils. They are pure plant essences that float on water after being distilled and act like oil.

An important question to ask is: where do essentials oils come from in nature? They are found in many species of leaves, flowers, trees, grasses, and fruits. They are found in the secretory system of plants, meaning the bark, leaves, seeds, petals, stems, and roots. An essential oil on average is about eighty times more potent than its dried form.

Essential oils are sourced from around the globe, including bergamot from Italy, sandalwood from Australia, lavender and rose from Bulgaria. When sourcing essential oils, the cardinal rule is that the plants are not harvested if they are not sustainable. Because terpenes and essential oils are a natural product and crops vary from year to year, you may on occasion find different aromas in the same fruit, spice, or herb. Essential oils are extracted from plant material in many different ways, including steam distillation, cold pressing, and solvent extraction.

There are many plants all around us with powerful properties waiting to be explored. Let's dive deeper into some everyday sources of essential oils for aromatherapy and learn where they are found in the world!

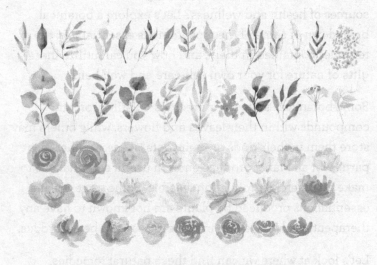

Different smelling flowers and herbs.

Botanical Breakdown

Humans discovered terpenes by studying plants. Plants have always contained great healing power, and their qualities have been studied and utilized via indigenous medicines since the beginning of time. How did our ancestors know that tea tree leaves, when distilled for their essential oil, would have antibacterial, anti-inflammatory, antiviral, and antifungal properties? It is incredible the number of remedies derived from one single refined essential oil. You might consider using tea tree oil to treat acne, dermatitis, athlete's foot, or even head lice.

So where are these amazing terpenes found in nature? And how can we harness our own foraging skills to find natural sources of health and wellness? Let's explore a botanical breakdown of some of the most famous essential oils, the terpenes contained in them, and how you can utilize these gifts of nature for your own self-care and well-being.

Some botanicals store their precious volatile aromatic compounds within their leaves and flowers, while others may store them in their rinds or their roots, seeds, or other plant parts. Not all plants produce enough useful essential oils to make commercial production feasible. Some terpenes and essential oils produced by plants are not known to have any therapeutic value and can in some cases even be hazardous.

Let's look at where we can find these natural remedies. Who knows—you may have some of them right in your own backyard!

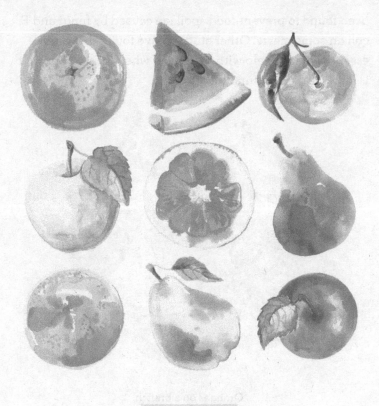

A set of fruits.

Orange

Mood lifter and pain reducer: orange essential oil is
extracted from the rind of the sweet orange (*Citrus × sinesis*).
This is done by cold pressing the rind, using pressure
to squeeze out the oils. Orange essential oils have been
study for their antimicrobial power and have been found
to aid in combating staph infections that are resistant to
pharmaceutical antibiotics. Orange essential oil was found
to kill bacteria without harming any human cells. It also has

been found to prevent food spoilage caused by fungi and E. coli on some meats. Other studies have found that orange essential oil can help with pain relief when inhaled orally. It is also used as a natural insecticide.

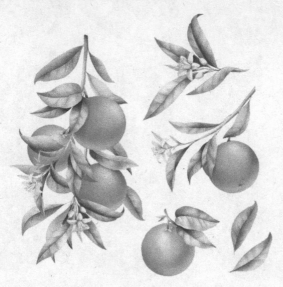

Oranges on a branch.

Tea Tree

Antibacterial action and reduces skin irritation: tea tree oil comes from the leaves of the tea tree (*Melaleuca alternifolia*), a small tree native to Queensland and New South Wales in Australia. Although this is known as a tea tree, don't confuse it with the plant that produces the leaves for teas one drinks, like black tea, green tea, and oolong. Tea tree oil has been used by native Australians for centuries. In traditional medicine, the leaves of the tea tree are crushed to extract the oils. Tea tree essential oil-laden steam or aroma is then inhaled to treat coughs and colds, or the essential oil is applied directly to the skin for healing (most often diluted—be careful). Tea tree oil contains a number of compounds including the terpene terpinen-4-ol, a terpene that has been shown to kill certain bacteria and fungi. Terpinen-4-ol also appears to increase white blood cell activity, which may help fight germs and other bacteria. The germ-fighting properties of tea tree oil make it a valued remedy for treating bacterial and fungal infections and promoting healing. Tea tree can be used as a natural hand sanitizer, insect repellent, or natural deodorant, using its antibacterial properties to control underarm odor. Tea tree oil can also be used as an antiseptic for minor cuts and scrapes—an antiseptic with the unique property of increasing wound healing abilities. To clean a wound with tea tree oil, first clean the cut thoroughly with plain soap and water, then mix one drop of tea tree oil with one teaspoon of coconut oil, apply a small amount of the mixture to the cut, and apply a bandage. Repeat this process daily until a scab has formed. Tea tree oil is a powerful tool for controlling skin issues like dandruff or psoriasis. Because of its strong bacteria killing properties, tea tree oil has many applications.

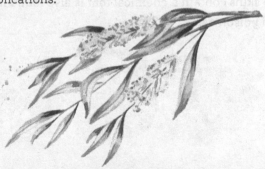

Tea tree branch.

Mango

Skin health: Mango is cultivated in more than one hundred countries and is one of the most consumed fruits in the world. Mangoes are packed with nutritious vitamins, minerals, antioxidants and terpenes, specifically myrcene. One cup of mango contains 67 percent of your daily vitamin C! Including mango in your diet is a great way to support your skin health as the high vitamin C helps with your skin's natural collagen production. The high antioxidant content helps prevent sun damage and premature aging. Rumour also has it that if you eat a mango before consuming cannabis, you will become more intoxicated because of the high concentration of myrcene. (Some evidence suggests this is true—we will discuss such effects further in the chapter titled "Cannabis and Terpenes" in the section on the entourage effect.) Mango oil is also extremely useful; it is generally derived from the skins, kernel and leaves of mangoes. Mango extracts contain a concentrated form of mangiferin that may have anticancer and antiaging benefits. A word of caution about mango: although uncommon, some people may experience an allergic reaction to mangoes. Mango skins contain a chemical that is also found in poison ivy and poison oak.

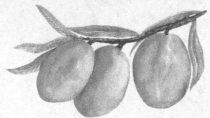
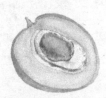

A mango branch and ripe mango fruits.

Hops

Relaxation and sleep aid: Hops are the female flower of the hop plant. They are used to flavor beverages like beer and for herbal medicines. The terpene humulene was discovered during research on cannabis. Researchers needed to find another plant that contained this new chemical compound they had discovered; they found that genetic match in *Humulus lupulus* (the scientific name for hops). Hops are a genetic cousin of cannabis, so it is no surprise that they are a sleep aid. The use of hops in ancient medicine in the East dates back to the emergence of Taoism about 2,500 years ago, while its use in Europe has been recorded since about the ninth century. Once hops became an ingredient important to beer manufacturers, scientists started studying the plant's effects on the body. The most prominent studies on hops suggest it may help improve sleep quality.

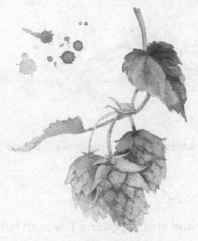

Hops on a vine.

Lavender

Relaxes and restores: The name *lavender* is derived from the Latin word *"lavare,"* which literally means to wash. The earliest recorded use of lavender oil was in ancient Egypt, where it was employed during the process of mummification. In later years BC, lavender became a bath additive in several regions, including ancient Greece, Rome, and Persia. These cultures believed that lavender helped purify the body and mind. Since ancient times, lavender has been used to aid with a plethora of mental health issues including stress, anxiety, and depression. It also aids with insomnia, headaches, nausea, and skin irritation. Today, lavender is most commonly used in aromatherapy. The fragrant essential oil of the lavender plant, featuring the terpene linalool, is known to promote calmness and wellness. This is why bubble bath is often scented with lavender.

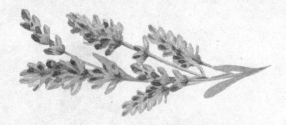

Lavender sprig with leaves and buds.

Mint Family

Boosts energy and aids digestion: The mint family of flowering plants (lamiaceae) comprises over seven thousand plant species, including oregano, basil, rosemary, lemon balm, and mint, which occurs in various types such as spearmint and peppermint. Plants in this family typically synthesize high concentrations of volatile and pleasantly odorous terpenes including menthol, menthone, isomene, caryophyllene, linalool, limonene, and terpineol.

When taken orally, menthol helps relieve gastrointestinal problems like indigestion, gas, and bloating. Menthol promotes the flow of bile to the duodenum where it assists digestion by facilitating the body breaking down fats more quickly. The high concentration of menthol found in the mint family is well-known and is used to treat an array of human disorders.

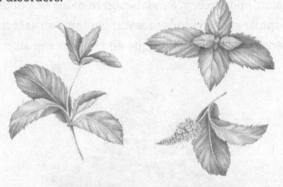

A collection of different mint plants.

Sandalwood

Healing: Sandalwood oil is found in many perfumes and air fresheners. It's a classic scent from a valuable tree. But the value of sandalwood goes beyond its smell; sandalwood offers many health benefits as well. Sandalwood oil comes from the wood and roots of the sandalwood tree (*Santalum*

album). The sandalwood tree is one of the most valuable trees in the world. Its products are used across the globe, and sandalwood oil is prized for its uses in traditional medicines. It is used to treat a variety of conditions including fighting bacteria, supporting wound healing, managing anxiety, and increasing alertness. Sandalwood oil has been used to treat the common cold, urinary tract infections, digestive problems, hemorrhoids, and mental health issues. Sandalwood's scent makes it a popular choice for aromatherapy and perfumes; in aromatherapy, sandalwood essential oils are diffused into the air to be inhaled, promoting better health outcomes in people with stress, depression, and anxiety. Sandalwood remains one of the most popular essential oils today. It contains an assortment of terpenes that create its unique and entrancing aroma.

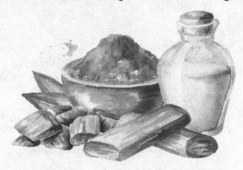

Sandalwood and sandalwood essential oil.

Bergamot

Skin and hair care: Bergamot oil is extracted from the rinds of the bergamot orange (*Citrus bergamia*). If you are a fan of Earl Grey tea, you've already enjoyed the distinctive taste of bergamot, which is used to flavor it. Bergamot trees can be found all over the world but gained prominence in the town of Bergamo in Southern Italy, which also gave bergamot its name. Bergamot oil is prized for its soothing scent, spicy taste, and medicinal properties, with a wide range of uses. You can use bergamot oil in a variety of applications from perfume and cologne to personal care and even flavoring food and drink. Bergamot is highly touted for its soothing use in aromatherapy. Several compounds in bergamot oil have antibacterial and anti-inflammatory properties. This makes bergamot oil effective for spot treatment of acne for people who do not have a sensitivity to its use on their skin. Its analgesic qualities make it an effective treatment against painful cysts. Try mixing bergamot oil into water when cleansing your face after testing for sensitivity on a small area first. Bergamot is great for your hair and can even aid in healing a sore scalp. A small 2015 study in Japan found that inhaled bergamot oil mixed with water vapor reduced feelings of anxiety and stress. The terpene linalool is found in abundance in bergamot and may be effective in destroying bacteria related to food-borne illness. A 2006 study found bergamot oil destroyed several strains of food-borne illness bacterium found on chicken skin and cabbage leaves.

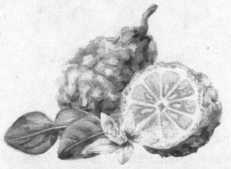

Bergamot fruit and bergamot flowers.

Rose

Pain reducing and antianxiety properties: poets and lovers have long sung the praises of the rose, but this flower is more than just a pretty array of fragrant petals. According to research, the essential oil derived from the rose plant has a wide range of potential benefits. Although a lot of the research is based on small trials, some clear physical and psychological benefits have emerged. In a 2015 study, children who inhaled rose oil saw a significant decrease in pain. Researchers believe that inhaling rose oil makes the brain release extra endorphins—naturally occurring feel-good hormones produced in the human body. Another study showed that massaging abdominal muscles with rose oil produced reductions in pain due to menstrual cramps. Rose oil has been shown to reduce blood pressure, heart rate, breathing rate, cortisol levels, and blood oxygen levels, all of the common symptoms of anxiety. Rose oil has also shown to reduce depressive symptoms and stimulate the sex drive.

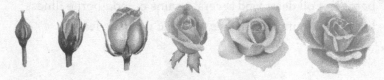

Blossoming rose in stages.

Chamomile

Digestion and wound healing: Chamomile is a flower species related to daisies. Chamomile oil is made from the flowers of the plant. There are two main types of chamomile, Roman and German, which vary slightly in appearance and chemical composition. The most researched active ingredient in chamomile is chamazulene, which is often grouped with sesquiterpenes, although, technically, it isn't one. Chamomile oil has been described in medical texts from ancient Egypt, Greece, and Rome. Over the centuries, it has been used to treat many things, including various types of digestive upset, such as indigestion, nausea, and gas. It has also been used for the treatment of ulcers, sores, and other wounds. Chamomile has long been thought of as a sleep aid. In a study of sixty seniors, participants who used chamomile extract twice daily reported better sleep. Chamomile tea is commercially available, or you can purchase the dried flowers in bulk and steep them in water to make your own more potent tea. Steam inhalation and vaporization of chamomile are also great ways to introduce the essential oil into your system.

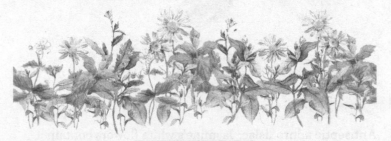

Chamomile plants.

Ylang ylang

Boosts mood and reduces depression: Ylang ylang is a yellow star-shaped flower that grows on the Carnaga tree. It is native to countries surrounding the Indian ocean like India, Australia, and the Philippines. Ylang ylang's heady, aromatic scent is fruity, flowery, and rich. Ylang ylang has a high concentration of the terpene linalool. There are many levels of distilled ylang ylang extract that vary in their intensity of aroma. It is used as a top note in many perfumes, including, most famously, Chanel No. 5. Ylang ylang has been proven to boost mood, reduce depression, alleviate anxiety, lower blood pressure, decrease heart rate, as well as repel flying insects and kill bug larvae. It is super easy to use ylang ylang: Try dabbing it on your wrist and smelling it, or, if you want to try your hand at making a natural bug spray, dilute it in water and spray yourself.

Ylang ylang yellow flowers.

Jasmine

Antiseptic aphrodisiac: Jasmine's white flowers contain a potent essential oil with many known benefits. The flower, which originated in Iran, is now grown in many tropical climates around the world. For centuries, jasmine has been popular for its sweet and romantic fragrance; it has been used in some of the world's best perfumes, including as a mid-tone in Chanel No. 5. Jasmine is a very popular ingredient in candy, baking, and alcohol. It is also used as a popular home remedy to treat many conditions from depression to infection but is best known as an aphrodisiac.

Jasmine's romantic scent has long been worn as a fragrance. In parts of India, jasmine flowers are included as décor at weddings and in newlyweds' bedrooms to set the mood. But there is very little scientific evidence to back up the claim that jasmine is an aphrodisiac. What we do know is that inhaling jasmine or using it in aromatherapy massage improves mood and has been reported to increase romantic and positive feelings. Jasmine is also an amazing antiseptic; it has been extensively studied and has been found to fight various bacteria. Jasmine oil may be effective in treating and preventing skin infections.

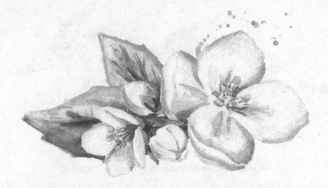

Sandalwood and sandalwood essential oil.

Lemon

Antimicrobial and anti-stress: Lemon peels are where you find a lemon's essential oils. The essential oil of lemons is a completely natural ingredient that has been used for centuries. It is packed with limonene and has an energizing and invigorating smell. Lemon essential oil is derived by cold pressing lemon peels. Lemon essential oils have actually been proven to yield the most significant stress reduction when inhaled, more than even other essential oils such as lavender and rose. It is also believed that the use of lemon in aromatherapy helps reduce nausea and vomiting. Lemon essential oil is great for killing harmful bacteria that grow on skin. It also has protective properties since it contains antioxidants that may brighten and preserve your skin. If you have acne, you may have already tried using lemon to clear your pores. If you are experiencing a cold or sore throat, try setting up a lemon essential oil diffuser; it could relax both your mind and the muscles in your sore throat.

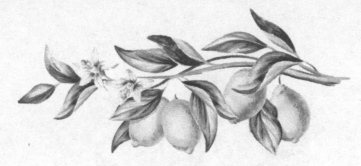

A lemon tree branch in bloom with fruit.

Cannabis

Physical and metaphysical well-being: The essential oils of cannabis are complex and abundant. Cannabis has evolved with complex terpenes and cannabinoids including THC & CBD which combine to give cannabis its antifungal and pest repellent properties. The essential oils of cannabis are contained within resin glands, each with a stem and a head, that sit all over the soft tissues of the cannabis plant. (When dry, this resin is commonly referred to as "the crystal"—a desirable feature found in abundance on high quality cannabis flowers.) The cannabis plant has been responsible for many breakthroughs in the study of terpenes. The cannabis plant possesses a potentially unlimited combination of terpenes. Cannabis breeders can create almost any kind of smell in the plant. Because of cannabis's past decades of prohibition, many plant breeders choose specifically fragrant plants that present the best smells and flavors, ranging from blueberry and lemon to diesel-filled cake. Cannabis genetics have been intentionally designed to yield the most and finest terpenes. Weed that actually smells like a raspberry lemonade smoothie or vanilla wedding cake is a reality. Some cannabis flowers have up to 5 percent terpene content by weight!

Most notably, cannabis produces an abundance of myrcene in broad leaf (indica) strains and limonene in narrow leaf (sativa) strains. Cannabis has long been prized for its medical effects and was regularly prescribed as medicine before the onset of prohibition in the 1920s. There are many well researched studies on the wide-ranging medical benefits of the cannabis plant. Cannabis and its abundant blend of terpenes and cannabinoids have long been used as a miracle drug for everything from countering anxiety to cancer suppression. Today, the cannabis plant has been legalized in thirty-six states and is medically available in fifteen; cannabis is now completely legal in Canada at the national level, with much of the rest of the world soon to follow.

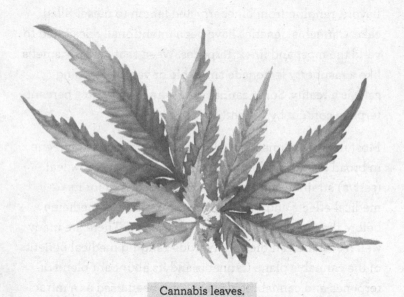

Cannabis leaves.

Terpenes and Aromatherapy

Aromatherapy is a holistic healing treatment modality that uses natural plant extracts to promote health and well-being. Sometimes aromatherapy is referred to as essential oil therapy. Once these oils have been extracted, the highly concentrated oils can be either inhaled or applied to the skin by various methods to increase both physical and emotional health.

Aromatherapy is thought of as both an art and a science. Recently, it has gained more recognition in the world of science and medicine. Essential oils and aromatherapy are a form of alternative medicine that employs plant extracts to support health and well-being. Medicinal claims surrounding essential oils are controversial and relatively little is yet known. Many animal trials have been done showing positive health benefits for many ailments, but very few human trials have been conducted. As our global populations search for ways to make our bodies healthier and more virus resistant, we will see more peer-reviewed studies being published proving the efficacy of essential oils as medicine for humans.

As people become more concerned with health and wellness in a time of pandemic, they are looking for natural solutions to help them stay healthy. Terpenes and essential oils have shown a multitude of positive benefits when vaporized in the air, from cleaning and cleansing the air around us to cleansing us from the inside when directly inhaled into our lungs.

Aromatherapy is a fantastic and positive way to lift your mood and immune system while enjoying a wonderful smelling aroma around you.

The term "aromatherapy" was coined by René-Maurice Gattefossé, a French perfumer and chemist, in a book he wrote in 1937, *Gattefossé's Aromatherapy*. Having discovered the miraculous healing power of lavender in treating burns, he went on to author a book discussing the use of essential oils as medical treatments.

Humans have used aromatherapy for thousands of years. People in ancient India, China, and Egypt, among other cultures, were known to add aromatic plants to balms, oils, and baths. These natural aromatics were used for medical and religious purposes. Ancient people understood that aromatic plants had both physical and psychological benefits when inhaled.

Aromatherapy works through the sense of smell (inhalation) and skin absorption. Here are some common methods for using aromatherapy products:

◆ Diffuser or vaporizer—used to vaporize and spread essential oils throughout a room.
◆ Aromatic spritzers—diluted essential oils in water sprayed in specific areas.
◆ Bath salts—Epsom salts blended with your favorite essential oils for relaxing therapeutic baths.
◆ Body oils, creams or lotions—add essential oils to unscented lotions or creams to unlock the healing benefits and aroma of the oils.
◆ Facial steams—adding essential oils to very hot water and inhaling while covering your head with a towel is great when feeling sick.
◆ Hot and cold compresses—add essential oils to the towel you are using as a compress to gain aromatherapeutic benefits.
◆ Clay masks—add essential oils into clay masks for their dermatological and aroma therapy benefits.

You can use any of these methods alone or in any combination as desired. Later in the book, we will discuss recipes and the best combinations of methods and terpenes for each desired effect.

There are hundreds of terpene and essential oil combinations on the market. Generally, people tend to use a combination of the most popular essential oils.

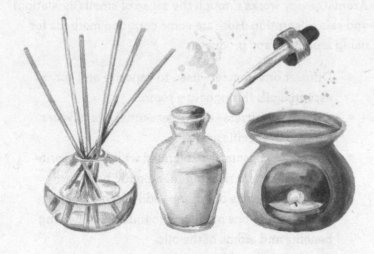

Essential oil diffusers.

Benefits of Aromatherapy

Aromatherapy has an extensive array of benefits, including:

- ◆ Pain management
- ◆ Alleviating inflammation
- ◆ Improving sleep quality
- ◆ Reducing stress, agitation, and anxiety
- ◆ Soothing sore joints
- ◆ Treating migraines and other headaches
- ◆ Alleviating the side effects of chemotherapy
- ◆ Fighting microbes of bacterial, viral and fungal origin
- ◆ Improving digestion
- ◆ Boosting immunity

Aromatherapy has the potential to treat many conditions. Though research is still ongoing, here are some conditions aromatherapy may treat successfully:

- **Asthma**—There is no cure for asthma, but many people have found relief from the symptoms of asthma by vaporizing oils like peppermint and eucalyptus. Both oils are known to be high in the terpene pinene. Pinene is often associated with relief of lung irritation.
- **Depression**—Depression affects many of us; it is estimated that around 7 percent of Americans will have a depressive episode in any given year. Using essential oils like lavender helps increase mood, decrease anxiety, lower stress levels, and promote relaxation—all amazing tools in combating depression.
- **Fatigue**—There have been many confirmed studies relating to essential oils and their effectiveness at decreasing fatigue and increasing focus. Lemon, orange, and peppermint essential oils have been the most widely researched oils; each shows positive effects for decreasing fatigue.
- **Insomnia**—Good sleep is essential for our bodies to function at their peak level. We have all experienced the stress of a bad night's sleep. A 2005 study at Wesleyan University assessed how lavender essential oils affected thirty-one young sleepers. Their research confirmed that vaporized lavender essential oil increased the amount of slow and deep wave sleep in participants. Participants noted feeling more vitality in the morning.
- **Alopecia**—Essential oils have been used for centuries to promote hair growth. The most well-known

aromatherapeutic oils to speed up hair growth are peppermint, lavender, and rosemary essential oils. Many other oils help hair growth as well, including lemongrass, cedarwood, and thyme.

◆ **Arthritis**—Arthritis gives rise to a number of painful physical symptoms, including pain, stiffness, and tenderness—and in addition, the chronic pain can be a constant emotional burden to the sufferer. Directly applying some essential oils to the skin can help a ton with inflammation from arthritis. No wonder every commercial pain-relieving cream has such a strong scent! Turmeric essential oil was shown to be 95 to 100 percent effective at preventing joint swelling in arthritic animals in a 2005 study from the University of Arizona.

◆ **Menstrual issues**—Since I am a man, I can not imagine how much having periods can suck. Studies show that cinnamon is the most effective essential oil for reducing inflammation and helping reduce symptoms of menstrual cramping. In a 2013 study at the Mansoura University, researchers concluded that women who received aromatherapy massages on the abdomen during menstruation reported less discomfort and pain. (Later in the book, we will learn how to make our own oils and lotions for massage.)

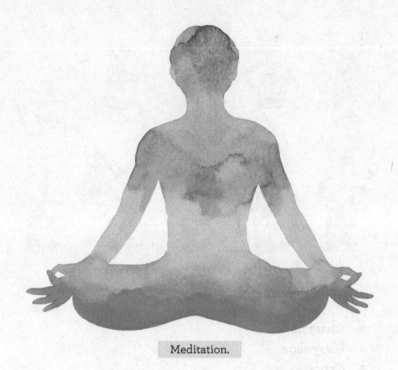

Meditation.

The Most Popular Essential Oils

You can use essential oils in so many ways! It's as easy as adding a few drops of essential oil to an existing body lotion. Try enhancing your facial toner, shampoo, or conditioner with your favorite essential oils.

According to the National Association for Holistic Aromatherapy, these are the most commonly used essential oils and terpenes.

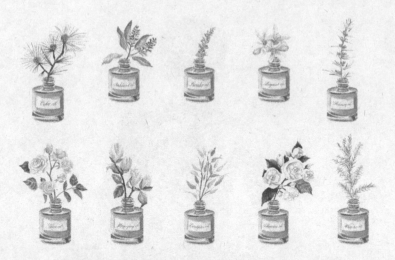

Different essential oils and herbs in aroma bottles.

- Chamomile
- Clary sage
- Cypress
- Eucalyptus
- Fennel
- Geranium
- Ginger
- Helichrysum
- Lavender
- Lemon
- Lemongrass
- Mandarin
- Neroli
- Patchouli
- Peppermint
- Rose

- Rosemary
- Tea tree
- Ylang ylang

This is a wonderful list that covers the most popular and useful essential oils. All of the listed essential oils are familiar to most of us and have proven benefits, aside from smelling amazing! The essential oils on the list can be found in most scented commercial beauty and dermatology products. Having the most common essential oils in your collection makes it easier to recreate recipes and aromas you may enjoy.

Storing your essential oils correctly is essential when building an essential oils collection. Remember oils do go bad with exposure to light and oxygen over time, so start with small quantities and make sure they are stored away from light and heat. Don't go overboard buying your first medicine cabinet of essential oil supplies!

What to Look for When Shopping for Essential Oils

Look for therapeutic grade essential oils. Therapeutic grade essential oils are the highest quality essential oil and can be used safely without worry. Therapeutic grade oils are pure and undiluted.

Be wary of marketing hype and claims. The Food and Drug Administration (FDA) doesn't regulate essential oils. Be wary of any oil that claims it can be used to treat or cure a specific condition. In the age of pandemic, I have seen many essential oils advertising as combatants or cures against COVID-19. Essential oils are a great tool for making positive impacts on your overall health and well-being but cannot cure or treat in full any medical condition.

Be wary of any essential oil claiming to treat a virus or disease. This author has seen some wild Covid cure claims by unknown companies.

Check the scientific name of the plant on the product label. This can help you make sure you're getting the type of essential oil you want.

Look for purity statements. You should be getting 100 percent essential oil. If the product is mixed with something else, the label should let you know.

Smell the product before purchasing it. If it doesn't smell like chamomile oil, as an example, don't buy it. The nose always knows. If something does not smell good or appealing to you, don't buy it. Commercial essential oils have been developed for the best-smelling aromas, so if it smells bad, it will never smell any better.

Look for dark colored bottles. Light can damage essential oils, so look for bottles that keep the light out.

Learn to determine quality by using your nose. Quality grading can be difficult if you are a beginner to essential oils as they will all smell particularly strong. Grading the quality of an essential oil is based on how potent the fragrance is.

Look for 100 percent non-GMO oils.

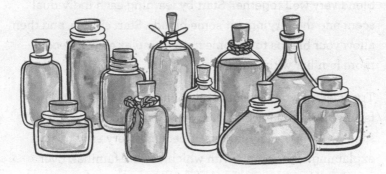

Essential oils.

Essential Oil Starter Set

Most starter sets of essential oil include six vials of essential oils, each containing ten ml. Ten ml of any essential oil is the perfect amount to test a particular oil. There are a plethora of essential oil starter kits available across the internet. As an initial investment for a six bottle set, I would look to spend from twenty to thirty-five dollars. There are many different options you can shop across the internet, or try finding a local fragrance and aromatherapy store.

These are the six starting essential oils I would recommend:

- Peppermint oil
- Orange oil
- Eucalyptus oil
- Lemon oil
- Tea tree oil
- Lavender oil

These scents are easily diffused or inhaled on their own and blend very well together. Start by learning each individual scent and then trying out some blends. Start simple, and then allow your blends to become more complex as you become more familiar with them.

Try smelling your essential oils blindfolded to become very familiar with their scents. Once you can recognize each scent without visual markers, it becomes very easy to start explaining other scents with which you are familiar. Ever wondered how a wine sommelier's description of a particular vintage rolls off the tongue so eloquently? It is a skill developed through blind tasting.

Blending essential oils can be tricky at first, but, with a basic understanding, you will be able to achieve your desired aromas. When starting out blending essential oils, it is easiest to do batch sizes in multiples of ten for easiest math. When making larger batches, a hundred drops is the normal starting amount. This is about one teaspoon of essential oil. Using one hundred drop batch sizes makes it easier when calculating dilution, adding your oils to a carrier oil for skin care, or combining oils into water for vaporization.

You should always dilute essential oils to a concentration of between 1 and 5 percent in a carrier oil; you can choose coconut oil or an unscented lotion for skin care, or dilute in water for vaporization. A couple drops of essential oils go a long way.

When combining essential oils, the most balanced blends will have top, middle, and base notes. Essential oils are made up of many different aromatic compounds including terpenes, alcohols, and esters. All of these individual aromatic compounds evaporate at different rates. A top note heavy oil is one whose aroma disappears quickly, while a base note tends to evaporate very slowly.

Top note essential oils	Middle note essential oils	Base note essential oils
quickest to evaporate	moderate rate of evaporation	slow to evaporate
strongest initial aroma, weakest aroma long term	weaker and less complex aromas than top notes, strong, lasting aroma	weakest initial aroma, aromas grow with strength after time, broad and heavy aromas
lemon, tea tree, grapefruit, peppermint, eucalyptus, chamomile	rose, mandarin orange, lavender, helichrysum	sandalwood, patchouli, cedarwood, myrrh, frankincense

Essential oils.

Blending Tips

Record your recipes and blending experiments in a notebook! You never know when you might strike gold!

Put labels on your bottles as you blend so you can easily replicate your successful blends or avoid recreating ones you don't enjoy.

Try peppermint with wild orange or tangerine for an uplifting and invigorating essential oil blend.

For a relaxing and calming blend, try blending lemon and lavender together.

When creating your own blends, think about aromas found in nature, like roots, woods, leaves, flowers, and fruits. Now, group two or three of these scent families together and select your essential oils to blend.

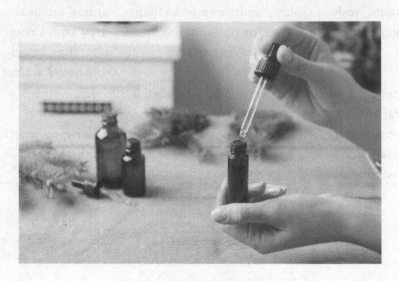

Blending oils in a bottle.

How to Use Terpenes and Essential Oils

We have learned about where we can find terpenes, and we have searched high and low to find the best essential oils. Now, how do we consume them? There are many applications for adding aromatherapy to your everyday life. Here are a few of the best (and my favorite) ways to consume terpenes and essential oils.

Vaporization

Vaporization of essential oils is one of their most enjoyable applications; it involves using one of a variety of devices to vaporize essential oils into the air that we breathe. When you vaporize essential oils, you not only have a pleasant aroma wafting in the air but get to have the beneficial therapeutic effects of the essential oils.

The most common way to vaporize essential oils is to add them to a vaporizer or diffuser. Essential oil vaporizers come in many different materials, ranging from terra-cotta or other types of ceramic to metal or even glass. These are made of two pieces, with the top part holding water and essential oils and the bottom housing a candle to generate heat.

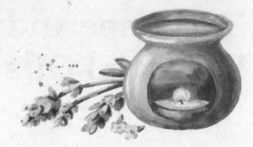

Essential oil aroma diffuser and lavender sprig.

Vapor therapy can also be as simple as placing a drop of essential oil on a handkerchief and inhaling.

When buying a vaporizer, look for one with a large top reservoir. The more water it is able to hold, the less often you will have to refill it. On average, you'll need to place about six to eight drops of essential oil into the water to be vaporized. As soon as the candle below starts to heat up the water, the essential oils are being vaporized and released into the air.

An alternative to a candle style diffuser is to use an electronic or ultrasonic diffuser. Electronic diffusers are easy to use, look cool, and are safe without the need to have an open flame burning.

Vaporization of essential oils forces their molecules to become airborne, which can benefit us in a couple of ways; the aromas trigger our limbic system through our sense of smell, and they are also absorbed through our lungs when we breathe, allowing the essential oils to enter the body directly.

Vaporizing essential oils has shown to help human health in a multitude of ways including easing respiratory tract problems, treating throat infections, relieving mental and physical fatigue, reducing tension and anxiety, and calming the nervous system.

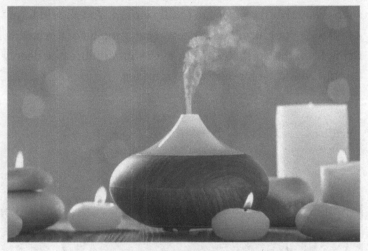

An essential oil vaporizer and candles.

Steam Inhalation

Steam and essential oils combined are a very potent way to treat some ailments, especially those of the upper respiratory tract, including the nose and sinuses. This treatment can be effective when you are suffering from a cold, wheezing in the chest or experiencing sinus discomfort.

This type of treatment should not be used for anyone who suffers from asthma.

Instructions for Steam Inhalation

Pour hot water into a bowl and add three drops of the essential oil you have selected. Place your head about twelve inches above the bowl and cover your head with a towel in such a way that the sides are totally closed. You should form a tent with your head and the towel catching all of the steam rising from the bowl. Keep your eyes shut and breathe deeply through you nose for one to two minutes.

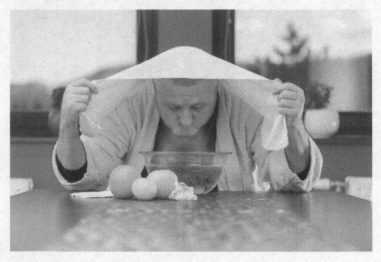

Man doing steam inhalation with oranges and ginger.

If at any point you feel the treatment is becoming too much for you, raise your head away from the bowl and lift the towel so fresh air comes in. Breathe through your mouth a couple of times, then try resuming the treatment. If at any time you should feel further discomfort, discontinue the treatment.

When using this treatment with children or elderly people, make sure their faces do not get too close to the water.

Here are some suggested essential oils for steam inhalation treatments:

- **Breathing difficulties**—cedarwood, eucalyptus, and pine (all high in the terpene pinene).
- **Bronchitis**—basil, cedarwood, clove, frankincense, pine, rosemary, thyme, and sandalwood.
- **Common Cold**—bay, black pepper, clove, ginger, myrrh, orange, pine, rosemary, and tea tree.
- **Cough**—cardamom, black pepper, peppermint, rosemary, and cedarwood.
- **Sinus**—lavender, peppermint, rosemary, basil, eucalyptus, and tea tree.

Oil and Lotions

There aren't many things more luxurious than using a nice essential oil-enhanced lotion on your skin. Why spend a fortune on commercial skin products when there are amazing all-natural products with wonderful scents that are far gentler on the skin?

A lot of people have a hard time starting out making their own essential oil blends because they don't know where to begin. It's actually very easy to make essential oil lotions once you begin doing it. I'm sure once you begin you will find it fun and exciting to experiment with different scents or to make creams for specific purposes, such as for daily skin care, acne, or to protect your skin from the cold winter air.

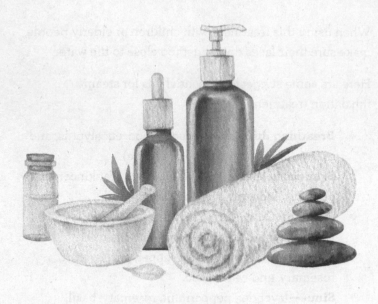

Spa items, lotion and essential oils.

Where to Start with Lotions

Carrier Oils

All essential oil lotions, creams, and salves begin with either
a single carrier oil or a blend of carrier oils. (To add cannabis
to your lotions, see the cannabis recipe section later in the
book for a basic cannabis infusion how-to.) For a thicker
cream or body butter, you would want to start with coconut
oil, for example. Coconut oil is stable at room temperature
but melts in your hands. You can make it creamier by mixing
one part coconut oil with another carrier oil like jojoba
or almond. Another great starting point for thick creams
is beeswax.

Other carrier oil options include:

- Grape-seed oil
- Jojoba oil
- Almond oil
- Argan oil
- Avocado oil
- Vegetable oil

You can get clues as to the quality of a carrier oil by where you purchased it and how much you paid for it. A single source coconut oil acquired at a farmers market may be of a higher quality then the cheapest store-bought option. Fats and oils of quality are generally not cheap.

The purpose of the carrier oil is to dilute the essential oils in the recipe, so they don't irritate your skin. Remember essential oils can cause allergic reactions when they come in contact with skin, so if you develop any redness or discomfort, discontinue use of that oil or blend. Essential oils do not work well with your skin unless diluted, sometimes to a concentration as low as 2 percent. That's just a couple drops per tablespoon of carrier oil.

When working with your essential oils, remember to handle them carefully and keep the bottles sealed while not in use. If you do spill essential oils on your skin, dilute them with vegetable oil and then gently rinse them off with warm soapy water.

Another reason that carrier oils are so important is that essential oils and terpenes are very volatile and evaporate rapidly. Without a carrier oil, the essential oil applied directly to the skin would never be able to penetrate deep enough to provide whatever benefit you are seeking.

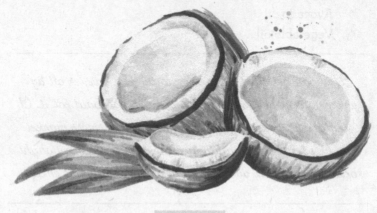

Coconut.

Making a Lotion

Now that we have covered carrier oils, we can get started! Combine your liquid essential oils with your beeswax and/or coconut oil. You may also want to add coconut butter or shea butter to improve the consistency of your finished product. Put all of your ingredients into a glass or metal bowl and place it over a pot of warm water (double boiler). The steam from the water will make the ingredients melt, making it possible to stir them all together easily.

Once the oils have reached a homogenized, liquid consistency, you can start adding in the "active ingredients." Vitamin E oil is a popular choice for lotions and skin care routines because it is an antioxidant and helps protect the skin against sun damage and other elements like cold and wind.

Some of my favorite essential oils to add to lotions are lavender, chamomile, sandalwood, ylang ylang, and tea tree. You do not need to use a lot of each oil. Remember just a few drops is plenty to give your lotion a beautiful scent and feel the therapeutic effects.

The type of essential oils you choose to use in your lotion can also depend on the purpose of use. For sports or exercise, peppermint and ginger are great to add for their cooling effects. Chamomile is calming for sensitive skin. Argan oil and patchouli are wonderful for antiaging face creams.

Aqueous vs Oil Lotions

The big difference between a lotion and a body butter is the amount of water in it. With most creams, more than half of the tub is water! When you are making homemade lotions, the problem with water is that it creates a breeding ground for mold and bacteria. This means if you'd like to keep the oil fresh, you will need some sort of preservative. Luckily some essential oils such as tea tree work wonderfully as preservatives.

A body butter is less likely to spoil quickly, but a lot of people don't like them because of the texture. Water-based oils are a good choice for those people. There are some active ingredients that work really well with water-based oils, including aloe juice, rose water, and witch hazel. If you can master a recipe that emulsifies water with oils, you will be in a good position to make any cosmetic product.

Carrier oils are packed with nutrients and antioxidants that can offer a ton of benefits for your skin. You may have heard oils are bad for your skin. Well, this isn't necessarily true. Some oils reduce inflammation and balance natural skin oils, preventing flare-ups, while other oils are great for eczema and dry skin.

To mix oils, including essential oils, with water, you will need an emulsifier. One great natural emulsifier is emulsifying wax made from wheat straw. You will need about 3 to 5 percent emulsifier for any recipe. (Coconut oil also works as an emulsifier.)

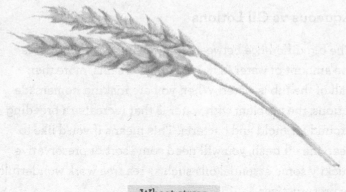

Wheat straw.

I usually don't add preservatives to my lotions, but if you would like yours to last more than a month, I would suggest using a natural preservative like rokonsal or leucidal in a proportion equal to 1 percent of the total volume of lotion.

When you first start making lotions and creams, start simple. Master a couple different recipes, and then start experimenting with different types of essential oils until you find something you love!

Using Terpenes for Physical and Emotional Well-Being

We have explored many ways we can find terpenes and essential oils in our daily lives and how they can be creatively utilized to better us. Since the beginning of time, humans and animals have turned to plants for their powerful healing properties. As of late, there have been great renewed interest in essential oil therapies. With increasing amounts of the global population affected by depression, anxiety, and diabetes, it is no wonder researchers and scientists are searching for sustainable and natural cures.

Herbs and essential oils have been used in medicine because of their biological properties, such as larvicidal action, analgesic and anti-inflammatory properties, antioxidant, fungicidal, and antitumor activities, and many more. Many essential oils exhibit antimicrobial properties, which are extremely important in various fields of science and industry, such as medicine, agriculture, and cosmetology.

Today there is freshly renewed interest in using essential oils and terpenes to improve physical and psychological well-being. A recent poll by *Insider* found that one in three Americans believes in the health benefits of essential oils and aromatherapy. Essential oils and terpenes are no longer merely a niche folk medicine but a strongly emerging alternative therapy with plenty of accredited research to support it.

Don't expect essential oils to be magical elixirs. They should never replace standard medical care. They can provide small benefits for individuals, but they should be seen as self-care life enhancers rather than medical treatments.

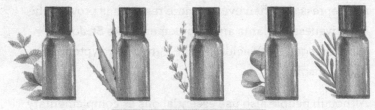

An array of essential oils.

Using Essential Oils to Help with Depression

Depression, a very common disorder today, is becoming a major health concern around the world. Today, depression affects over 350 million people across the globe. Depression is the leading cause of disability worldwide. It can affect the way you feel, think, and act, and although depression is a mood disorder, it can present both physical and emotional symptoms. From anxiety to restlessness, sadness, poor concentration, and difficulty sleeping, depression can manifest itself differently in different people. The social and economic impacts depression is having on society have led researchers to investigate further remedies for the condition.

We know that prescription drugs often have negative and unintended side effects. Depression medications, while commonly prescribed, can cause unfortunate physical and mental interactions. Terpenes have quickly become a very important compound in natural and synthetic antidepressant designs and drug development.

Today more people are choosing naturally based antidepressants than ever as more research is proving the effectiveness of plants and supplements like St. John's Wort, omega-3 fatty acids, 5-HTP (5-hydroxytryptophan), and cannabis.

Although people also use essential oils as complementary treatments for many conditions including depression, it is important to note that essential oils are not a cure for depression. They are a drug-free option that may help treat some of the symptoms.

To inhale essential oils, dab a couple drops on your wrist and breathe in the scent. Also try dabbing the essential oils into a cotton ball or handkerchief and inhaling.

Research suggests that these are the best essential oils to vaporize and inhale to help with depression symptoms:

- **Lavender**—Lavender's floral and earthy scent is valued for its calming and relaxing effects. It helps relieve anxiety, decrease stress, promote relaxation, and improve mood.
- **Wild Ginger**—It is thought that wild ginger may activate serotonin receptors, lifting the mood and slowing the release of stress hormones.
- **Bergamot**—Bergamot has been known to greatly reduce anxiety in hospital outpatients who took part in aromatherapy research studies. The scent of bergamot is uplifting and calming. Although anxiety and depression are different disorders, they often show up at the same time, so it is good to take note of antianxiety essential oils.
- **Cannabis**—Cannabis has been evaluated for years as an aid to treating depression. Researchers have shown that cannabis may be most beneficial in restoring balance in the human endocannabinoid system. Our endocannabinoid system is a system of receptors that has effects on our mood, appetite, and physical functions. The endocannabinoid system is the key to cannabis's medical benefits.

Terpenes and essential oils' activity are enhanced when inhaled as they can have a direct impact on the central nervous system.

Today we have more research and products available to us than ever before to help combat depression. Using terpenes and essential oils is a wonderful way to reduce your symptoms of depression with natural supplements that smell delicious and are proven to work when combating such conditions.

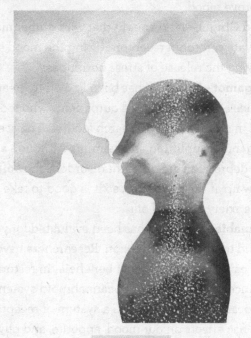

Inhalation.

Before you decide to take any supplements for anxiety, depression, or insomnia, consider the following:

- ◆ **Medication isn't always the answer.** Review the lifestyle habits that influence your sleep: make sure you take no caffeine late in the day, have a regular sleep schedule, exercise regularly, and wind down an hour or two before bed. Try cognitive behavioral therapy. Replace worries about not sleeping with positive thoughts that may be more effective and safer than medications or herbal supplements for insomnia. Consider that there may be important underlying causes, such as sleep apnea or restless leg syndrome, which require medical evaluation.

◆ **Product claims may be misleading.** Don't just rely on a product's biased marketing. Search for honest, research-based information to evaluate a product's claims. The National Institutes of Health are good places to start.

◆ **Talk to your doctor.** If you are taking medication, it is always safest to talk to your doctor to make sure any natural supplements won't interact with other medications or supplements you're taking and that they are safe to take with any medical conditions you have.

Bottom line, chronic insomnia indicates a problem, such as poor sleep habits or a medical or psychological condition. Consider getting an evaluation at a sleep medicine center.

Using Terpenes for Antiviral Properties

Including SARS & COVID-19 (SARS-CoV-2)

When we are sick, we boost our self-care regimen as we wait for the infection to run its course. Increasing water intake and rest is crucial to beating a bug quickly. How can we use terpenes' natural virucidal (virus killing) properties to help prevent sickness as well as treat ourselves better when we become sick?

The emergence of never-before-seen viral diseases such as COVID-19 has necessitated research on the effectiveness of new antiviral agents, such as terpenes. As a result, scientists have learned that monoterpenes are effective antiviral agents. Terpenes are the major components of plant essential oils. Plants use them in their own defenses against natural bacteria, viruses, and pests.

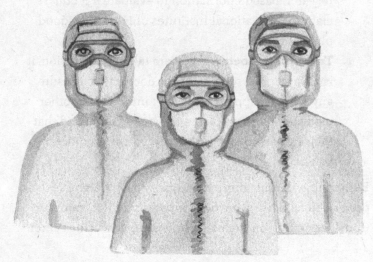

People in antiviral suits.

In studies posted by the US National Library of Medicine (ncbi.nih.gov), one study evaluated the antiviral activity of essential oils extracted from various South American plants. The oils were tested against three major human viruses—herpes simplex virus (HSV1), the dengue virus, and the Junin virus. The oils that were highest in limonene, pinene, caryophyllene, and camphor proved to have antiviral properties. Other studies have researched essential oils' effectiveness for treating serious respiratory maladies like Severe Acute Respiratory Syndrome or SARS-CoV-2 (COVID-19). Many plants have similar terpene combinations in their essential oils, and these blends could be a solution for problems shared universally. Another study found that while essential oils do not directly combat COVID-19, however they have shown that they may act synergistically with other antiviral agents, making them more effective. Essential oils also provided relief from the symptoms of COVID-19.

The terpene shown to have the strongest virucidal properties is pinene. Researchers are working on synthesizing and creating terpenes from fungal forms. The fungus that produces pinene is easily grown and readily harnessed for its presumed antiviral qualities and UV protective properties. Terpene production from fungi could lead to very cost-effective terpenes with very limited labour needed in production, making them a viable medicine commercially.

The possibility of being able to grow antiviral terpenes from fungal sources is a massive opportunity for naturally sourced, low-cost medicines. As we look toward a more sustainable future, these fungal sources may provide affordable medicines that are not generally available today. We don't yet know exactly what the far-reaching opportunities will be for terpenes in relation to COVID-19 or other respiratory viruses, but there is some promising validity to what has been proven already with the antiviral and virucidal properties of essential oil compounds in relation to some respiratory viruses.

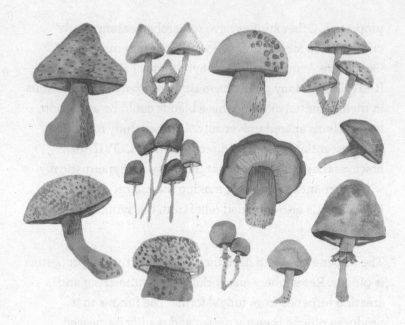

Mushrooms.

If you are feeling a little sick at present and would like to harness the powers of essential oils, I would recommend inhalation. Inhaling different essential oils comes with a combination of benefits. Feel free to sniff your essential oils directly, add them to a handkerchief or cotton ball, add them to bath water, put them in a diffuser, or try steaming them for steam inhalation.

There are many essential oils, and they all carry different benefits. Each one has specific beneficial properties depending on its application. For example, the effects of peppermint and menthol are known to work better when topically applied and rubbed on the chest then when they are diffused.

- ◆ Lemon oil—promotes steady breathing and clears nasal passages
- ◆ Lavender oil—relieves headaches, stress, and fatigue
- ◆ Peppermint oil—clears sinuses, reduces coughing, and soothes throat infections
- ◆ Thyme oil—strong antibacterial properties help fight respiratory infections
- ◆ Eucalyptus oil—reduces fevers and fights viruses
- ◆ Tea tree oil—fights infections and inhibits bacteria growth
- ◆ Chamomile oil—relieves cold and flu symptoms
- ◆ Clove oil—has antiviral and antifungal properties
- ◆ Rosemary oil—cleans surfaces and air of bacteria and viruses[1]
- ◆ Cinnamon oil—can clean surfaces and air[2]

Remember to always dilute your essential oils with a carrier oil if you are using them topically.

---

1   Rosemary oil is considered useful for cleaning surfaces and air of bacteria and viruses; however, for safety's sake, further steps should be taken to ensure disinfection. Before using essential oils to clean surfaces, CDC and WHO approved disinfectants, such as rubbing alcohol at 70–90 percent strength, should be used to clean the area. Where highly contagious airborne viruses may be present, masks should be worn, and measures such as strategic ventilation, filters, and/or UV light may help to make spaces safer in combination with masks. The right essential oil can provide a nice final step, cleansing, adding aroma, and helping set a positive mood.

2   Cinnamon oil: See above.

In a 2010 study that looked at a commercial essential oil blend of clove, wild orange, and cinnamon oils, its application reduced in vitro viral particles by 90 percent. The oil blend also proved to decrease infection.

While essential oils are great for helping fight viruses like colds and flu, you should not rely on them as your only treatment. There are many over-the-counter medications that are effective and can decrease your recovery time.

Always make sure to talk to your doctor if you are feeling unwell.

Do not eat essential oils, and do not use concentrated amounts of essential oils. Always dilute essential oils.

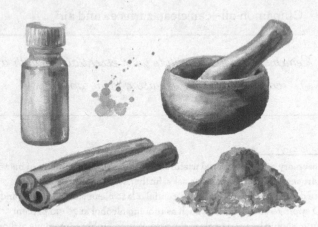

Cinnamon and cinnamon essential oil.

Diabetes and Essential Oils

Diabetes is one the most prevalent diseases affecting children and adults across the world. The social and economic burden of diabetes continues to grow and is expected to continue to rise rapidly in developing countries. In North America, diabetes is a leading cause of visual impairment, limb amputation, kidney diseases, heart disease, and death.

There are two types of diabetes—Type 1, in which the body's immune system acts against insulin-producing organs, and Type 2, in which either the insulin produced cannot be used by the body or production is not sufficient.

Several medications are available for diabetes, but their use may be restricted by harmful side effects. Essential oils do not treat diabetes but can help with many of the peripheral complications that come with diabetes. Essential oils are great for combating infections which people with diabetes may be more susceptible to.

As mentioned, there is no medical human trial evidence to support using essential oils for diabetes, but it may be used to treat complications of diabetes like gastrointestinal issues and weight gain.

Essential oils should be used with caution in conjunction with treatments recommended by your physician. Essential oils should be inhaled or diluted in a carrier oil and applied to the skin. Do not swallow essential oils.

Here are some of the most effective essential oils for helping with diabetes:

- **Cinnamon**—In a 2013 study on pubmed.gov, researchers found that people with prediabetes and diabetes who ate cinnamon experienced a decrease in blood pressure. Although the study focused on the spice and not the essential oil, one could make the inference that cinnamon essential oil would likely have the same effects. More research is needed to build on previous limited studies, so do not rely on cinnamon as a medication to control your blood pressure.

- **Rosehip**—Rosehip essential oil is known to help with weight management. Researchers conducted a twelve-week study of thirty-two participants with a body mass index between twenty-five and twenty-nine. Participants received either rosehip extract or a placebo. At the end of the study, those who used rosehip extract had a significantly larger decrease in abdominal fat as well as body fat and their body mass index had decreased.

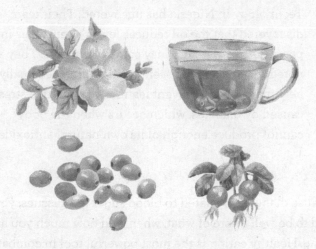

Rosehip and rosehip tea.

- **Coriander seed oil**—Better known as cilantro, the coriander seed is a great remedy for digestive issues like gas, diarrhea, and indigestion. Coriander seed oil has also been shown to help reduce blood sugar levels in diabetic rats in a 2009 study from the Azad University. Researchers noted that cells in the pancreas were more active after using coriander seed oil. This may help increase insulin levels and decrease blood sugar.
- **Lemon balm**—Lemon balm essential oil may help people with high blood sugar levels. Researchers have found that lemon balm oil helps encourage cells to consume glucose. Human studies have not been done yet, but early research suggests it may be beneficial.
- **Clove bud essential oil**—Clove bud oil may play a major role in preventing and managing Type 2 diabetes, as research from the Federal University of

Technology in Nigeria has uncovered. Their team discovered that the oil reduces levels of enzymes in the pancreas in a way that may combat diabetes. They also noted that clove bud essential oil might specifically help manage and prevent features of oxidative stress caused by diabetes, which occurs when the body cannot produce enough of its own natural antioxidants.

Nutrition and Exercise

Because diabetes is related to blood sugar level issues, you need to be well aware of what, when, and how much you are eating. Healthy eating is the most powerful tool in combating diabetes. Limiting your sugar intake and eating clean healthy food are extremely powerful tools. People with diabetes often find benefit in talking and working with a nutritionist to ensure they are getting the nutrients needed without excess sugar.

Physical activity helps control blood sugar levels and blood pressure levels. It is recommended everyone get thirty minutes of physical activity daily.

Do not ignore your doctor's recommendations or prescribed medications for treating diabetes.

Essential oils can be great tools for helping with the stress and anxiety surrounding diabetes. They are best used vaporized or diluted in carrier oil and are never ingested orally. In the next chapter, we will explore how you can use terpenes and essential oils in your life. A calming bath or infused massage oil is a wonderful way to relax and benefit from the amazing effects of aromatherapy.

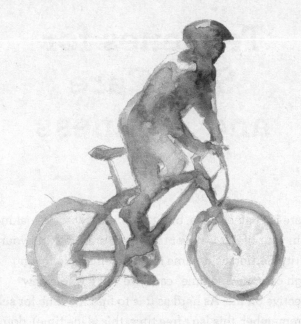

Biking.

Terpenes for Self-Care and Wellness

Self-care isn't a new idea, but it is definitely worth making a habit in your life! It is never too late to start making yourself a priority. Setting aside time for yourself and following through on your "me time" can give you a whole new perspective on life. As hard as it is to find the time for self-care (remember, this isn't free time, this is me time), doing so pays off by preparing you to tackle obstacles in your life with a clearer head and fuller heart. Put yourself first and try some of these self-care routines with your favorite essential oils.

Focusing on yourself creates an opportunity to refocus and reenergize. Serving others brings a wealth of benefits, but we can't be great for other people if we are not great to ourselves first. You should enjoy an afternoon nap and a long essential oil enriched bath. You deserve it.

There will always be something else to add to your to-do list. It's okay to leave some items off now and again to take a break. Try taking time for yourself every day and do something you love. Once self-care becomes a habit for you, you may find it easier to make your needs a priority in other aspects of your life.

How to Use Terpenes in Baths

Soaking in a warm bath is therapeutic on so many levels. Hot baths are instantly relaxing. A hot bath is likely to soothe even the sorest of muscles and joints. Adding terpenes and essential oils to your bath can be a beautiful addition as they release even more benefits, making your bath an even more luxurious experience.

Here are some amazing ways to enhance your bath using some of the essential oils we have already talked about:

- **Lavender**—Lavender is extremely popular as a bath addition due to its gentle scent and effect on people's mood. Lavender is often used to promote relaxation and balance, supporting a more restful sleep. Lavender is also known to relieve pain and inflammation. Try a few drops in your next bath.
- **Lemon oil**—Lemon and other citrus fruit essential oils have all been shown to have benefits when used for aromatherapy. Just remember lemon oil makes your skin very photosensitive, so don't go right out in the sun after using it.
- **Eucalyptus**—Eucalyptus has very strong sharp scent that can open up your nasal passages in a way similar to menthol. The scent is sometimes too strong for people, so try adding some sweet orange, geranium, or sandalwood to tone it down.

Other popular bath additions are:

- **Roman chamomile**—Used by the ancient Romans to give courage during war, this beautiful aroma is often found in tea but works great in baths as well. Chamomile oil is often found in perfume and face creams because of its nourishing effect on the skin and calming effect on the mind and body.

- **Frankincense**—Frankincense is known as the king of essential oils. This powerful essential oil is revered for its ability to beautify and rejuvenate skin when applied topically. Considered one of the most prized and valuable possessions of Biblical times, frankincense was esteemed by ancient civilizations and has been used in the most sacred practices. Remember frankincense was a gift presented to Christ after his birth. The aroma makes you feel peaceful and relaxed.

- **Ylang ylang**—Ylang ylang is has been used for centuries for its wonderful scent and nourishing properties. You'll often find it employed in commercial hair and skin products for its scent and nourishing qualities. Ylang ylang's aroma is known to lessen tension and stress; it blends well with geranium, bergamot, and grapefruit.

Citrus oils include grapefruit, lemon, and bergamot essential oil. Bright citrus fruits are great for aromatherapy, with uplifting and invigorating aromas known to make people feel energized. Grapefruit is renowned for its cleansing and purifying properties and is frequently used in skin care products as a tonic for clear and healthy skin.

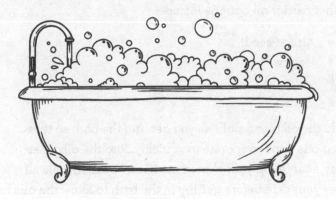

A bubbling bath.

Make Your Own Essential Oil Bath Mixes

When making essential oil mixes for the bath, it is easiest to start with one kind of essential oil and add it to a carrier oil before introducing it to your bath. Diluting the essential oil in the carrier oil is important so that the concentrated oils will not irritate your skin if they stick to you when floating in the water.

Here's how to mix your own blend of essential oils for baths:

A dilution rate of 1 to 4 percent is recommended for essential oils you want to use in your bath. It is advisable to use vegetable oil as the carrier oil.

- 2 teaspoons carrier oil (10 milliliters)
- 3 drops essential oil = 1 percent
- 6 drops essential oils = 2 percent
- 9 drops essential oils = 3 percent

Other carrier oil options include:

◆ Grape-seed
◆ Jojoba
◆ Almond
◆ Argan

Add the oil blend right as you get into the bath so that your oils don't evaporate too quickly. Rub the oils in as they float up on your skin in the bath, or rub the oils all over your skin before getting in the bath to allow the oils to deeply penetrate.

These are some wonderful oil blends to try in your bath. Quantities given are for one bath:

◆ Relaxation: 3 drops of lavender + 3 drops of fennel + 3 drops of wild orange
◆ Soothing: 3 drops of lavender + 3 drops of chamomile + 2 drops of cedarwood + 1 drop of lemongrass
◆ Awake & attentive: 3 drops of peppermint + 3 drops of lavender + 3 drops of grapefruit + 2 drops of lemon grass
◆ Sweet dreams: 3 drops of lavender + 3 drops of orange + 2 drops of chamomile + 1 drop of sandalwood
◆ Calm: 4 drops of myrrh + 3 drops of chamomile + 4 drops of orangs + 3 drops of lemon
◆ Alert: 4 drops of peppermint + 4 drops of grapefruit + 2 drops of rosemary
◆ Skin toning: 4 drops of myrrh + 4 drops of patchouli + 2 drops of geranium

There aren't many combinations of essential oils that don't work, to be honest. If it smells appealing to you, then it probably blends well. You can easily open two jars of essentials oils and smell them together to see if they synergize. Just remember to always dilute your essential oils and be careful not to use too much—a little goes a long way.

You can also try infusing any of these combinations of essential oils into Epsom salts if you prefer. Just put your Epsom salts in a container with a lid, add your oils, and shake. They will store for a month, but it's easiest to make it by the single-bath portion.

Bubble Bath

Using castile soap (which is amazingly versatile), dilute your diluted essential oil into a small amount of liquid soap in a small bottle. Shake the bottle vigorously, then add it as the bath water is running—again, mixing it in just as you're about to enter the bath.

Use Essential Oils in the Shower

You don't have to have a bathtub to use essential oils in your routine. In the shower, put 3 to 5 drops of essential oil on the upper wall or outer edge of your shower; the hot water will diffuse the scent as you bathe.

Make the Best of Your Bath

If you have the time when taking a bath, make a special day or evening of it. Enjoy a hot cup of chamomile, lavender, or peppermint tea with honey. Take your time, any amount of time.

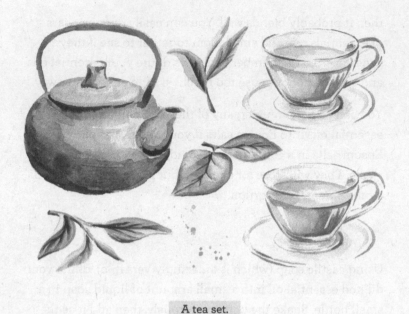

A tea set.

Aromatherapy Massage and Massage Oils

Massages are absolutely amazing. How do we improve something that's already so pleasurable? Let's add essential oils to our massage. We know that essential oils and aromatherapy are fantastic for many different purposes, from relaxants to aphrodisiacs. Massage is wonderful for relaxation, pain management, and improved mood. It only makes sense for these two to go hand in hand.

Applying essential oils directly to the skin is a fantastic way for them to be directly absorbed into the body quickly.

Aromatherapy is often added to a traditional massage session as an extra service. The massage therapist may diffuse oils in the room or add a few drops of essential oils to the massage oils.

Tips for Aromatherapy Massage

◆ Decide whether you want to diffuse the essential oil into the air or apply it directly to the skin mixed with the massage oil.

◆ Choose an essential oil based on your needs and desires; for example, lavender is great for relaxing, whereas citrus is a wonderful mood elevator.

◆ Drink lots of water before and after getting massaged.

◆ Take a warm shower after your massage session to help remove any excess oils.

Remember some essential oils and aromatherapies can irritate people with allergies or asthma. If you are being massaged and feel any discomfort, it is your job to speak up. Because massages are intended to be relaxing experiences, it is rare for your massage therapist to ask you questions.

Some of the most popular oils for aromatherapy massage are:

◆ Bergamot
◆ Cedarwood
◆ Chamomile
◆ Eucalyptus
◆ Geranium
◆ Ginger
◆ Lavender
◆ Lemon
◆ Orange
◆ Peppermint
◆ Tea tree

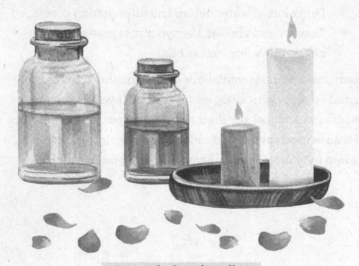

Essential oils and candles.

Self-care is so important in our lives. We very quickly forget that such priorities matter. Taking a moment to have a bath or massage yourself are freeing moments that we all deserve.

Here are some other great ways to practice self-care in your daily life:

- Take a walk with no destination in mind
- Start your morning with food you truly love
- Meditate
- Stretch
- Drink lots of water
- Keep a journal, and feel free to write anything—journaling helps free the mind

Another fantastic self-care ritual I practice daily is consuming cannabis. Cannabis helps with my physical and metaphysical well-being. Beyond the benefits of cannabis' rich abundance of terpenes and cannabinoids, simply taking time to focus on its aromas and flavors while rolling and smoking it is extremely valuable for daily pause and self-reflection.

Setting Intentions

Intention has the power to change your life. Let me explain.

What does intention mean, and what gives it power? "The power of intention" is a hot phrase these days, for good reason. I truly believe the power of intention can change your life.

To put it plainly, setting an intention is activating our willingness to try and experience new things. If you go out in the day without any set intention and have not envisioned any kind of manifestation idea of how you'd like the day to go, it is as if you are getting in a car and driving to nowhere in particular. That can be great, but sometimes we want to go somewhere. The power of setting intention helps you get there.

Intention is so significant because it slowly shows you how truly powerful you are as a human. Oftentimes we just let the day, week, or month slip away. When you set your intentions, you are activating your willingness to receive and manifest what you intend to attract in your life.

Setting intentions is not only for the tangible; it's not about physical things. Being mindful about your spirit, body, and mind can be extremely powerful.

Your intentions do not have to be large and broad. Try making them realistic throughout every day: "I want to have a great morning meeting with my team," or "I am excited for a new work opportunity to become my responsibility."

Once you have your intention in mind, it's time to tell the universe. How do you do that? For me I scream it out loud, really loud, multiple times, although this method is definitely not for everyone. Others would suggest spending a night in the bath, nourishing and caring for yourself, taking some time to journal when you are nice and relaxed, and trying to set some intentions for the next week, month, or year.

We are constantly seeking or wanting more. It is important to reflect on what we have when setting intentions and finding moments of gratitude. When you can be happy in what you already have, accomplishing simpler things feels much more pleasurable. When you are constantly wanting, you are in a state of need or scarcity.

While setting intentions sounds easy enough, it is important to remind yourself of them, daily as well as weekly. Try succeeding with your smaller day-to-day intentions and visiting your large ones once a week.

Try starting out each day by placing your hand on your heart, breathing deeply, and sending love to yourself and the day. Then set your intentions for that day.

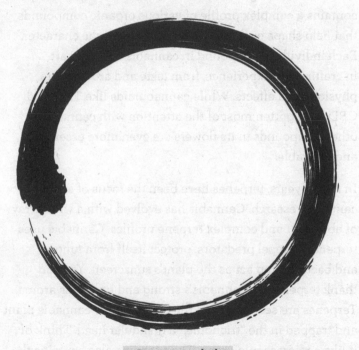

An enso symbol.

Cannabis and Terpenes

Cannabis has a long and interesting history. It has only been in the last decade that we have really seen cannabis normalization begin to come to fruition. The cannabis plant contains a complex profile of various organic compounds that help shape each individual strain's unique character. Each individual compound in cannabis does its part in crafting the experience, from taste and aroma to its physiological effects. While cannabinoids like THC and CBD have gotten most of the attention with cannabis, other compounds in its flowers are even more essential and desirable.

In recent years, terpenes have been the focus of a lot of cannabis research. Cannabis has evolved with a wide array of abundant and complex terpene profiles. Cannabis uses terpenes to repel predators, protect itself from fungus and bacteria, and act as the plant's sunscreen. You can thank terpenes for cannabis's strong and unctuous aroma. Terpenes are secreted from the glands of the cannabis plant and trapped in the "trichome," a glandular head. Think of it like a microscopic grape. The trichome also contains the biochemicals that have intoxicating and medical properties within cannabis; these are known as cannabinoids.

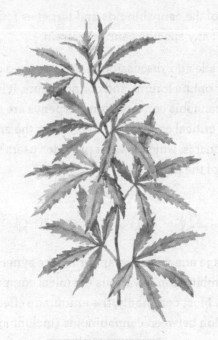

A cannabis plant.

As with many other aspects of the cannabis plant, there are still scores of questions relating to terpenes. The most common question pondered is just how many terpenes are present in cannabis? Today, over one hundred different terpenes have been identified in the cannabis plant!

The popularity of terpenes in cannabis as a topic of discussion exploded in 2012 when cannabis extracts started becoming popular. As cannabinoids and terpenes have been isolated from cannabis using solvent based extraction and distillation, cannabis terpenes have become much more refined, without all of the organic plant matter they were formerly attached to. A refined cannabis extract is the truest expression of the cannabinoids and terpenes found in the trichomes of any specific cannabis strain.

While a decade ago, discussion of terpenes and cannabis was reserved for online forums and connoisseurs, it is now a vital part of the cannabis conversation. Terpenes are regarded as the most critical component to creating the entourage effect of cannabis, which is what provides users the entire experience of the plant.

The Entourage Effect

The entourage effect is a metaphor for the synergistic effects from the combination of various chemical compounds found in cannabis. Most commonly, the entourage effect refers to the interaction between cannabinoids (including THC and CBD) and terpenes. Terpenes have been described as the "color" of cannabis. What does that mean? If we visualize a coloring book, we see black lines on white paper. Similarly, let's think of THC and CBD as those uncolored pictures— they create an image, yes, but one that is two-dimensional and without depth. Now add color to this picture; let's pick three colors. Imagine a child has colored in the picture with those three colors. Again, it's still two-dimensional, but it's changed into something a little more interesting. Now think of complex terpenes as the work of a professional artist. The picture has now become a piece of art unfathomable to the average human. Those three colors (or terpenes) have painted depth and complexity into it and added an entirely new dimension to the experience.

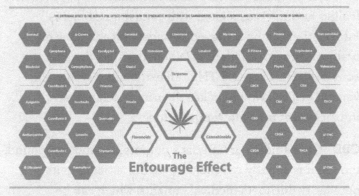

Entourage effect.

Before we take a deep dive into the entourage effect, let's go over some cannabis terminology.

Cannabinoids—We have talked about THC (tetrahydrocannabinol) and CBD (cannabidiol), but you may be surprised to know that these are only two of over 120 cannabinoids that have been recognized in cannabis today.

Cannabinoids interact with our bodies' endocannabinoid system (or ECS), a system composed of chemical messengers (endocannabinoids)and binding sites (receptors) located throughout the human body which regulate functions like appetite ("the munchies"), sleep, and pain. Every human has an ECS, just as we have a cardiovascular system or respiratory system regardless of whether we have ever consumed cannabis or not.

THC—Tetrahydrocannabinol, or THC, is the part of the cannabis plant responsible for the intoxicating psychoactive feeling or "high" associated with cannabis. Cannabis intoxication can be achieved by ingesting cannabis either orally or through inhalation. When ingested, the liver converts THC to 11-OH-THC, an extremely psychedelic version of THC which makes the user much more intoxicated at much lower quantities.

CBD—Cannabidiol, or CBD, is a nonintoxicating compound, though it is slightly psychoactive. CBD is rising in its popularity due to its medical benefits, which can be experienced without having to become intoxicated. CBD is the second most common compound in cannabis and is highly prevalent in hemp (a cousin to cannabis). Hemp plants must contain under 0.3 percent THC, but some strains have been found to contain up to 20 percent CBD!

THC & CBD.

How does it work? We know that cannabinoids and terpenes each produce certain effects on their own. But what happens when you mix cannabinoids and terpenes together in one inhaled experience? Since every terpene is unique in its chemical composition, each one offers something different in terms of effects. Most cannabis strains contain a variety of terpenes, making it nearly impossible to ascertain which cannabinoid and terpene pairings elicit a terpene entourage effect. With that in mind, research into terpenes provides some clues.

For example, neurologist and cannabis expert Dr. Ethan Russo contends, "Data would support the hypothesis that myrcene is a prominent sedative terpenoid in cannabis, and combined with THC, may produce the 'couchlock' phenomenon of certain chemotypes."

So, if THC + myrcene = a sedative cannabis intoxication, what other terpene entourage effects are possible?

As research into the entourage effect is still in its infancy, only time will tell. But it's entirely possible that in the future, instead of classifying strains by physical characteristics (i.e., sativa versus indica), we will instead think of each cannabis strain in terms of its chemotype or chemical profile—a much more accurate predictor of the strain's effects.

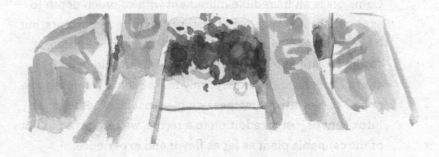

Rolling a joint.

Cannabis, Canapés, Cocktails (Plus Teas and More!)

Cannabis has many positive benefits for both your physical and metaphysical well-being. As cannabis legalization becomes a reality in more places in the world, we are finally able to utilize the amazing medicinal properties of this plant. Cannabis can be utilized in so many more ways than just by smoking it, and we are now seeing consumption of cannabis in food and beverage normalized at more and more dinner tables. The end of global cannabis prohibition is near, and it is very exciting to see.

Cannabis is an incredible ingredient with so much depth to explore. It is not only one of history's favorite intoxicants, but it is also packed with terpenes! With thousands of different strains of cannabis now being bred for their unique and alluring smells and flavors, it only makes sense for us to look at how to elevate our recipes using cannabis. Whether as an intoxicant or just an addition to a recipe, we can get a ton out of the cannabis plant as far as flavor and experience.

To get the active ingredients out of our cannabis, we will need to learn about a process called decarboxylation. Decarboxylation, or "decarbing," is a method of removing the acidic molecule or the "A" from THC-A. Cannabis in its raw form is hardly psychoactive at all. It is not until heat and time are applied to the equation that we can unlock cannabis's psychoactive effects. Cannabis cannot get you high until it is heated.

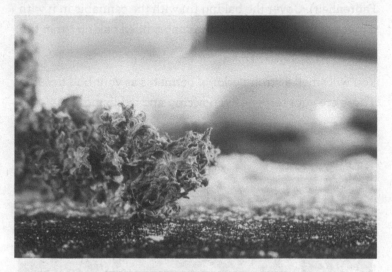

Cannabis bud and an egg yolk.

How to Decarboxylate Cannabis

The process of decarbing is much easier then saying the actual word "decarboxylation." As mentioned before, all you need to decarb your cannabis to unlock its psychoactive potential is heat and time. I will explain two very basic methods of decarbing. There are lots of fancy machines that will now do the decarbing for you, but at its most basic, all you need for the process is an oven or a warm pot of water.

The Oven Method

Place your cannabis in a small baking tin. You can separate your cannabis into smaller pea to popcorn size pieces. Warm your oven to its lowest temperature (200 to 250 degrees Fahrenheit). Cover the baking tin with the cannabis in it with a piece of tin foil. Place your cannabis filled baking tin in the oven for 45 minutes.

You will smell a strong odor of cannabis as your bud decarbs. These are your terpenes vaporizing and oxidizing.

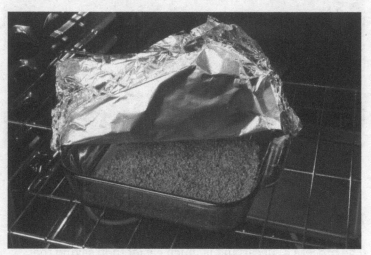

Cannabis being decarboxylated in the oven.

The Sous Vide Method

Place your cannabis into a freezer bag or vacuum seal bag. Warm a pot of water on your stove top to somewhere between 200 and 250 degrees Fahrenheit (medium low heat). Place the sealed bag containing your cannabis into the hot water for 45 minutes to fully decarb. If you have a sous vide machine, that will work the best for keeping the water temperature consistent. The sous vide method is much better at containing smell and preserving terpenes then the oven method.

Understanding and Calculating Cannabis Dosage

Deciphering cannabis measurements can seem quite daunting at first. With units of weight from ounces to grams as well as THC percentages to consider in purchasing decisions, it seems very confusing. But I promise you it isn't.

Visiting a cannabis dispensary for the first time can feel overwhelming. Cannabis flower weight and THC dosing can be confusing, even for seasoned consumers. Many of us grew up purchasing cannabis outside of a regulated system, never quite understanding exactly how much cannabinoids were in the product.

Now, when you walk into a dispensary, the budtender will probably ask you if you have any favorite terpenes or aromas you'd like in your cannabis. As we have learned, cannabis can present many different combinations of aromas from its natural terpenes and essential oils. By exploring familiar smells like lemon or blueberry, we are able to find cannabis strains that naturally taste and smell like things we desire.

With such a wide array of cannabis strains out there, it is impossible to understand dosage without knowing the exact weight and cannabinoid content of your cannabis.

Here are some helpful abbreviations and conversions that we will use shortly to calculate dosing:

> Milligrams = mg
>
> Grams= g
>
> Ounces = oz
>
> Pound = lb
>
> 1,000 mg = 1 g
>
> 1,000 g= 1 kilogram (kg)
>
> 16 oz = 1 pound (lb)

Fun fact: The weight of one cubic centimeter of water is one gram!

Understanding THC Percentages

When you buy cannabis flower from a dispensary, you will notice every strain is labeled with a THC content expressed as a percentage. To accurately figure out your dosage, we will use the THC percentage and the weight of the cannabis flower to determine how many milligrams of THC are in each edible.

Tip: If you are not purchasing your cannabis from a regulated source, there is no way to guarantee THC percentage.

We measure THC in milligrams (mg), so first we need to convert our flower weight to milligrams.

1 g = 1,000 mg

Then we measure the percentage of THC in the flower and calculate its weight in milligrams. Let's calculate the milligrams of THC for one gram of cannabis flower labeled as containing 15 percent THC.

1,000 mg x 0.15 = 150 mg of THC

Theoretically, you would have 150 milligrams of active THC in the gram of cannabis.

Now that you understand how to calculate the amount of THC in your cannabis flower, you can easily determine individual doses if you want to make edibles. Let's use the cannabis math from above and figure out the potency of each dose for a batch of brownies.

We will use 3.5 grams of cannabis, so given the 15 percent THC cannabis in our example, we will have 525 mg of active THC for our brownies. We will infuse the 525 mg of THC into one cup of butter. (15 percent THC = 150 mg of THC per gram of cannabis flower; 150 mg multiplied by 3.5 = 525 mg of THC in one cup of butter). We will therefore use a whole cup of butter for 24 servings.

525 mg ÷ 24 brownies = 21.88 mg of THC per brownie.

21.88 mg per brownie is a good size dose, one which should be taken with caution. A beginner dose should be 10 mg of THC to start, or even as little as 5 mg THC if the person is inexperienced with cannabis, very slender, or tends to be sensitive to medicines. An expert dose can be as much as 100 mg or more.

Basic Cannabis Infusion

Let me explain how to simply infuse butter and oil. Butter and oil are the two most versatile ingredients in cooking. Almost everything you can cook needs them, and they are almost guaranteed to make anything taste better.

Whether you are baking or making coleslaw, with this infusion method, you will be a master of the cannabis pantry.

Infusing cannabis is really just as simple as decarboxylating it. You need three things:

◆ Decarbed cannabis.
◆ A carrier fat (various plant and vegetable oils or milk fat).
◆ A vessel to heat the cannabis and carrier for 20 to 30 minutes. Use a crockpot or a pot on your stove top.

To infuse your oil or fat, bring it to a warm simmer and place your cannabis in it. Slightly agitate it every 5 minutes for 20 to 30 minutes. Then strain the cannabis plant material out using cheesecloth and discard the cannabis. All the active cannabinoids (including both THC and CBD) are now in your oil! Let it air and cool, then bottle and store in the fridge or pantry.

Your new cannabis infused oil has the same shelf life as it did before you added the cannabis to it! The shelf life of olive oil is around eighteen to twenty-four months.

These are some great carrier oils and fats to infuse and stock in your pantry:

- Olive oil
- Butter
- Coconut oil
- Avocado oil
- Grape-seed oil
- Walnut oil
- Dairy cream

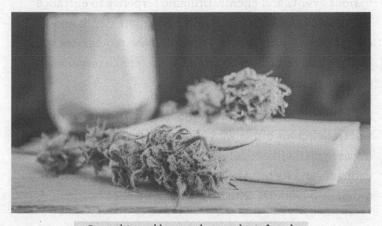

Cannabis and butter about to be infused.

How Much Cannabis Can You Infuse into an Oil?

The theoretical limit of cannabis infusion into any of the carriers mentioned above is about four grams of cannabis per quarter cup of oil. This means you could make an extremely potent oil using very small amounts of the carrier (58 mg per teaspoon); you could have upwards of 700 mg of cannabinoids in one quarter cup of oil.

I would advise caution when considering preparing an oil this strong, though. It's quite rare that anyone would want such a large dose. It is much easier to utilize infusions at a potency of around 5 mg per milliliter.

Terpene Enhanced Cocktail Recipes

I've invented all of the following cocktails over the years for various events and clients. Utilizing terpenes to entrance the senses is an incredible way to add more depth and complexity to your drinks. Through these recipes, we will explore how to burn, mist, muddle, and shake terpenes into our beverages.

All of these beverages can be made without alcohol, and each will be delicious either way. I have added a suggested spirit in case you do like to imbibe. We will also explore how to use cannabis and its terpenes to create alluring, intoxicating, and aromatic beverages with and without alcohol.

Set Your Intention

It is always appropriate to set your intention when creating anything. Remember that we are humans with the ability to create and enhance. We should put our truest feelings forward when creating anything; your intention will be returned to you by your creation.

Before beginning, try saying this mantra out loud:

"I am filled with love and positive intention; I have the power to create."

Infusing Alcohol or Simple Syrup

Creating infusions is much simpler and less daunting than one might at first imagine. To make infusions, you really only need two things: heat and time.

If you are looking to unlock the flavors and intoxicating effects of cannabis, this process becomes a little bit more complex, since you have to include the added step of decarboxylation.

Infusing anything is as simple as placing what you would like to infuse into the medium it will be infused into. In this section, we will look at a lot of different infused syrups. These syrups all start with the same base: simple syrup made of two parts sugar to one part water.

If you'd like to prepare an infusion using alcohol, again, simply add the desired material to be infused into the spirit. Generally neutral spirits like vodka are used to showcase the flavors of the infusion, but any spirit can be used. To speed up the process of infusion, use very low heat to draw flavors out more quickly. You can do this by placing your alcohol in a mason jar and then in a water bath or double boiler on an electric stove top at 160 degrees Fahrenheit. Let your decarboxylated cannabis steep for 15 minutes, strain, and enjoy. Make certain to only use alcohol meant for human consumption, since it is not safe to drink isopropyl or rubbing alcohol.

Caution: Never heat alcohol on any type of open flame, including a stove top. Do not overheat. Be sure the room is well ventilated as alcohol vapors can be produced; such vapors can be flammable as well as hazardous to breathe.

Alcohol evaporates at 172 degrees Fahrenheit, so you will only need to have your decarboxylated cannabis in the alcohol mixture for 15 minutes at 160 degrees Fahrenheit for full infusion.

The Linalool Sour

I love a good sour! The dancing acidity, the frothy egg white, the complex aroma—everything layers together so well, yet it's something so simple. Simple and delicious is always one of the hardest things to master, but once you do, a new world emerges. In my experience, the trick to a great sour is a very frothy egg white! For this drink, you will need to pre-froth your egg white vigorously. While frothing your egg white, to work on your shaking technique as you will need to go on shaking for about thirty seconds straight. Now that you are prepped with the fundamentals, here is what you will need:

Bar Tools Needed

◆ Mixing glass and shaker tin (or try using a mason jar if you don't have a bar set)

Glassware

◆ Coupe glass

Ingredients

◆ 1 egg white, vigorously shaken
◆ 1½ oz lavender syrup
◆ ½ oz lemon juice
◆ 1 oz lime juice
◆ Ice
◆ Linalool liquid terpene (True Terpenes brand recommended)
◆ Optional spirit: 1 oz Tanqueray gin

Instructions

1. Crack egg into shaker tin and shake vigorously for at least 30 seconds.
2. Combine lavender syrup, lemon juice, and lime juice with shaken egg white.
3. Ice and shake, shake, shake for 12 seconds.
4. Double strain into a coupe glass. (To double strain, first strain through a mesh strainer, then strain through a finer mesh strainer.)
5. Garnish with a sprig of fresh lavender or dried lavender flowers; add 3 dashes of linalool terpenes on foam.

Lavender syrup is made by adding dried lavender to warm simple syrup and steeping for one hour to infuse the flavor.

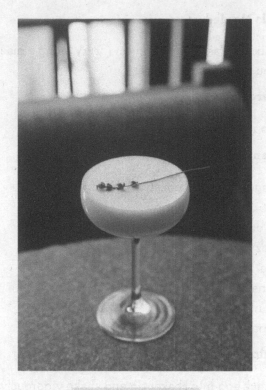

Lavender sour cocktail.

Ghost Train Haze

Acid! But not LSD! Ghost train haze is a citrus bomb. Perfect for hot summer nights, late afternoons, or anytime you are thirsty. Terpinolene and limonene dominate this fruit forward cocktail. Like a little bit of bubble? Try it in a Collins glass with some soda also!

Bar Tools Needed

- Mixing glass & shaker tin (try using a mason jar if you don't have a bar set)
- Atomizer (for spray mist)

Glassware

- Coupe glass or Collins glass

Ingredients

- ½ oz lime juice
- ½ oz lemon juice
- 1 oz grapefruit juice
- 1 oz orange juice
- Orange bitters
- Serrano Sour Diesel Hot Sauce (or Cholula)
- Tajin spice
- Salt
- Ice
- Optional booze: 1 oz Mezcal

Instructions

1. Combine lime juice, lemon juice, grapefruit juice, and orange juice in mixing glass. Add a small dash of Serrano Sour Diesel Hot Sauce or Cholula hot sauce and a tiny pinch of salt.
2. Ice and shake, shake, shake for 12 seconds.
3. Use a lime wedge to moisten the rim of the rocks glass and roll half of the rim in the Tajin spice.
4. Add ice to the glass and strain drink over top of the fresh ice.

5. Mist the glass with 2 sprays of orange bitters slightly diluted with water (The Haze).

The recipe for Serrano Sour Diesel hot sauce can be found on my YouTube channel, *The Cannabis Sommelier*. Just look for the "How to Make a 'Ghost Train Haze' cocktail" video.

To mist the orange bitters, you will need a misting bottle.

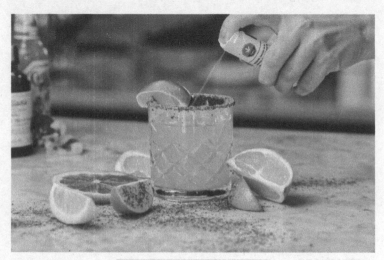

Ghost train haze cocktail.

Cold Lavender & Fog

I love London fog lattes! They are so entrancingly delicious and complex. Bergamot always makes me feel so warm. That slight hint of citrus combined with vanilla and warm milk is just perfect almost anytime. I thought about how I could have a London fog latte in a cocktail setting, and this is what I came up with! Lavender and bergamot are the stars of this cocktail.

Glassware

- Collins Glass

Ingredients

- 1 tablespoon loose Earl Grey tea, or 1 tea bag
- ½ teaspoon dried lavender flowers, plus extra for garnish
- 4 oz boiling water
- 1 oz lavender simple syrup
- ½ teaspoon pure vanilla extract
- ¼ cup nut milk (cashew milk or almond milk)
- Ice
- Optional liqueur: 1 oz Amaro

Instructions

1. Bring water to a boil.
2. Place the loose Earl Grey tea and dried lavender into a loose-leaf tea pot or a tea ball infuser. (See notes for tea bag method.) Pour half a cup of boiling water over the tea leaves and steep for 10 minutes.
3. Fill a Collins glass with ice. Strain the hot tea over the ice, leaving some space in the glass. Add the lavender simple syrup, vanilla extract, and nut milk, then stir. Taste for sweetness and add another drop or two of simple syrup if needed. Garnish with a sprig of fresh lavender or lavender leaves. Drink immediately.

To brew with a tea bag, place the tea bag and lavender leaves into a mug, then pour the water over. Steep, then remove the tea bag. Strain out the lavender blossoms using a small strainer.

Lavender syrup is made by adding dried lavender to warm simple syrup and steeping for one hour to infuse the flavor.

The Best Damn Moscow Mule

I love Moscow mules! The spice of the ginger and the acid of fresh lime play so well together. If you use a naturally flavored ginger beer, you can really unlock the potential of this amazing drink! For this Moscow Mule, we will make our own ginger syrup to unlock the healing powers of ginger. Ginger is incredibly powerful tool in aiding with digestion. This super spicy ginger syrup that is the center of this drink may just become a new staple in your refrigerator for other concoctions. Ginger has a blend of lesser-known terpenes that make up its alluring scent.

Bar tools needed

- Bar spoon (or any spoon, in a pinch)

Glassware

- Copper mug

Ingredients

- 2–3 oz ginger syrup
- Juice of ½ a fresh lime, or 1 oz of lime juice
- Club soda
- Ice
- Mint sprig (for garnish)
- Optional spirit: 1 oz vodka

Instructions

1. Add 2-3 ounces of ginger syrup to a copper mug. You may like it more or less spicy, so adjust the amount of syrup to your personal preference. Make sure to try it both ways!
2. Slice a lime and squeeze the juice of half the lime into the mug.
3. Ice the mug all the way to the top.
4. Add club soda to the lime juice and ice and stir ingredients together.
5. Garnish with a sprig of mint for aromatics.

To make spicy ginger syrup: Thinly slice a very large chunk of ginger and add it to a pot containing warm simple syrup. Add 10 to 15 black peppercorns. Leave the warm syrup with the ginger and pepper on very low heat for 2 hours.

To make ginger candy: Strain your ginger syrup and bottle. Take the thinly sliced pieces of ginger and lay them flat on a baking sheet. Turn your oven down to its lowest setting and slowly dry the ginger pieces, which have been coated and soaked in sugar while in the simple syrup.

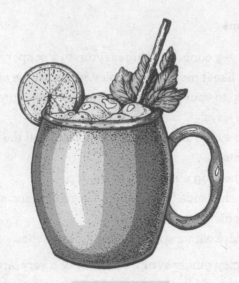

Moscow mule.

Cold Apple Pie

I wanted a drink that tasted like I was eating cold apple pie—so, I made it! Seriously though, who doesn't love cold apple pie!? Something about the pie spice and the snap of the apple always brings me to a perfect place and moment. The cold apple pie is also breakfast for the next morning—a perfect segue from one perfect moment to the next. Also, um, excuse me, yes, you can eat pie for breakfast! My mother told me so!

Bar Tools Needed

♦ Mixing beaker or shaker tin

Glassware

♦ Short rocks glass

Ingredients

- 1 oz chai and apple pie spice syrup
- ½ oz lemon juice
- 2 dashes of angostura bitters
- 5 oz cold pressed apple juice (a bit more than half a cup)
- Apple pie spice and sugar (to dip the rim of the glass)
- Apple slice for garnish
- Optional spirit: 1 oz bourbon

Instructions

Before you begin:

- To make the dry mixture for dipping the glass rim, add 3 parts white sugar to 1 part apple pie spice mix.
- To make the chai and apple pie spice syrup, stir 1 tablespoon of apple pie spice mix into warm simple syrup along with a chai tea bag to steep for 1 hour on very low heat.

1. Ice your mixing beaker, then add all the wet ingredients to the glass.
2. Stir for 20 seconds for proper dilution.
3. Take your rocks glass, wet the rim with a lemon wedge or lemon juice, and dip the rim into your sugar and dry apple pie spice mixture.
4. Add fresh ice to the glass and fill to the top of the glass with the mixture from the beaker.
5. Garnish with a thin apple slice in the glass, placed along the edge so it is visible.

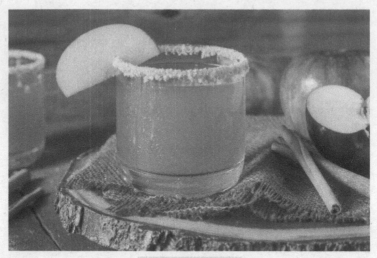

Cold Apple Pie.

There is no limit to what you can create in a cocktail! The flavors that you love and enjoy can easily be combined to create exciting new flavors. Remember to include three things when creating your own cocktail recipes: Sweet + acid + ice usually equals a wonderful drink so long as everything is in the right proportions. Try making your favorite classic cocktail and upgrading your bar skills! My favorite classic limonene forward cocktail is a shaken lime margarita. If you'd like to find more of my cocktail recipes online, check out my YouTube channel, *The Cannabis Sommelier*.

Cannabis and Herbal Teas

Tea is such a beautifully basic thing, one that unlocks so many incredible and complex aromas and flavors. Tea is prepared by pouring hot or boiling water over leaves, flowers, and/or roots and steeping these botanical materials. After water, tea is the second most consumed beverage in the world. There are myriad kinds of tea, from green tea to chamomile. Teas can be sweet, nutty, floral, bitter, astringent, alluring, and complex.

Tea originated in the regions known today as Northeast India and Myanmar. It has been used as a medicinal beverage by many cultures dating back to the third century AD. The term "herbal tea" refers to teas made with infusions of fruits, leaves, rosehips, chamomile, etc. Tea itself can only be made from the tea plant (*Camellia sinensis*).

Drinking tea often has a calming or relaxing effect. Pairing that with a blend of herbal infusions makes it the perfect vessel to enhance, producing a terpene filled beverage with multiple beneficial effects.

Cannabis tea, like other forms of cannabis edibles, is a great way to consume cannabis without having to smoke it.

There are a few main ways you could make a cannabis tea:

◆ Infuse your tea with decarboxylated dry cannabis flower (see section on decarboxylation).
◆ Mix a cannabis infused carrier oil into a latte type coffee or foamed milk beverage.
◆ Add a cannabis tincture to a tea.

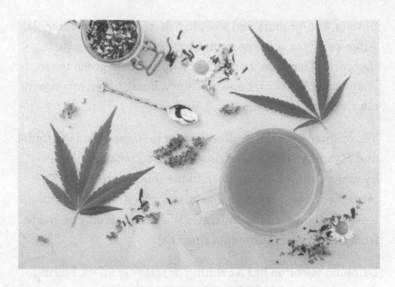

Cannabis tea and herbs.

How long does cannabis tea take to kick in?

Cannabis tea is processed just like any cannabis edible in your body, meaning it has to pass through your stomach and then be metabolized by your liver. This means it can take from one to two hours to feel the effect of your cannabis tea. Unlike smoking, where you are likely to feel the effects instantly, tea takes some time to kick in, and the intoxication may come on slowly.

A word of advice: When drinking cannabis tea, start low and go slow. Don't overdo your dosage. Don't drink multiple cups quickly back-to-back. Drink a cup and wait. You can always go back for more later.

Here are some basic cannabis tea recipes. The first recipe, which uses chamomile and lavender, can be reinterpreted in a variety of ways. Simply switch it up using your flower or tea of choice along with ground, decarboxylated cannabis.

Lavender Chamomile Cannabis Tea

This deliciously relaxing recipe can be upgraded with many different additions, from lemon and ginger to peppermint.

As far as dosage, it is recommended to use between 10 and 50 mg of THC or 0.1 to 0.3 of a gram of decarboxylated cannabis flower.

Tools Needed

- ◆ Tea infuser

Ingredients

- ◆ 2 teaspoons of dried chamomile
- ◆ 2 teaspoons of dried lavender
- ◆ Honey (optional)
- ◆ Milk or coconut milk (optional)
- ◆ 0.1 to 0.3 grams of decarboxylated cannabis

Instructions

1. Add all of the dried flowers (lavender, chamomile, and cannabis) to a tea infuser, cover, and steep in hot water for 5 to 10 minutes.
2. Pour and enjoy! It's as simple as that. You can choose to add milk or honey to your tea.

Try mixing up your tea flowers next time! Maybe use some fresh ginger or lemon peel in your blend for added flavor.

Remember, peppermint is great for digestion and blends wonderfully with these ingredients.

Cannabis Chai Latte

A latte is traditionally a coffee drink with espresso and steamed milk, but using just the steamed milk with different tea blends can yield an incredible depth of flavor and fantastic cannabis infusions.

Let's consider chai tea, or rather masala spice tea. It is a delicious tea blend brimming with aromatic spices and steeped tea leaves. Adding another natural ingredient like cannabis is a no-brainer. Chai tea's unique flavors are packed full of terpenes and essential oils with powerful natural nutrition benefits, so it's no surprise that it is popular with those creating anti-inflammatory diets.

Chai tea is an ancient blend derived from Northern India and Chinese remedies. The blends were often used in traditional medicines to heal mild coughs, infections, and other chronic disorders. Chai tea's recipe has taken many different forms as it has been passed down through the generations but is still a revered antidote for headaches and fatigue in India.

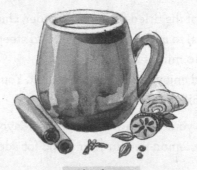

Chai latte.

Traditional chai spices include:

- Ginger
- Clove
- Nutmeg
- Cardamom
- Cinnamon
- Black pepper
- Vanilla bean
- Star anise
- Fennel seeds

Many of these spices are known to alleviate anxiety and promote good health.

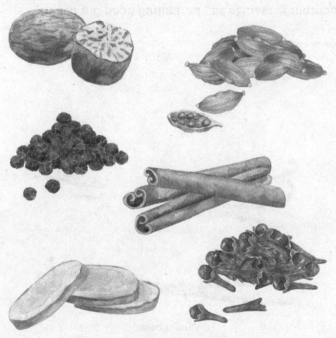

Masala chai.

The power of a cannabis infused chai latte is in the synergistic effects between the herbs and spices. If you are making your own chai tea blend, here is a little more on the health benefits its ingredients offer.

Health Benefits of Vanilla Bean

Vanilla, which gives most people's favorite ice cream its flavor, is thought of as merely a sweetener and flavoring agent. But with high levels of magnesium, calcium, and vitamins A and D, real vanilla bean extract is a potent source of nutrients. The sweet aroma of vanilla has been known to alleviate stress and anxiety, and the vanilla bean is also great for curbing cravings and promoting good gut health.

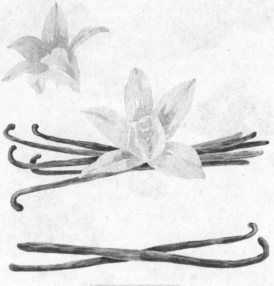

Vanilla bean.

Health Benefits of Black Pepper

Pepper may be the most widely used spice in the world! But for some naturopathic practitioners, it is more than just a culinary spice; black pepper has antimicrobial, anti-inflammatory, and antibacterial properties. A truism in the cannabis world is if you are feeling too high (intoxicated), you should chew black peppercorns to release the intense amounts of beta-caryophyllene and pinene terpenes found inside, as this is known to bring some people back to a better regulated state. Aside from bringing you back from too much cannabis, black pepper is also known to improve metabolism, fight bacterial infections, and control blood sugar and cholesterol levels.

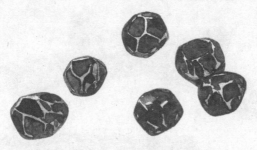

Black peppercorns.

Health Benefits of Cardamom

Cardamom is an ingredient found in many ancient Tibetan medicinal remedies. The spice is known to have antibacterial, anti-inflammatory, and antimicrobial properties, making cardamom a great spice for supporting your immune system. Cardamom is known to detoxify the body, improve blood circulation, improve metabolism and digestion, and combat allergies and respiratory disorders.

Health Benefits of Cinnamon

Cinnamon is extracted from the bark of the cinnamon tree. Cinnamon bark is packed with essential oils as well as with terpenes like cinnamaldehyde and eugenol. It is these phytochemicals that make cinnamon such a powerful ingredient There are many different types of commercially available cinnamon, with the most common being cassia cinnamon. Cinnamon is a superfood known for its antibacterial, antifungal, antidiabetic, and antioxidant properties.

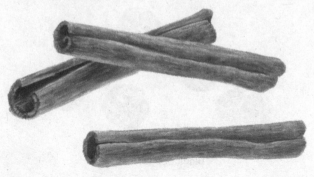

Cinnamon.

Health Benefits of Clove

Clove comes from the flowered buds of the clove tree, also sometimes called the "tropical myrtle" tree. The clove tree gives off a distinct fragrance, and its flowering buds are full of vitamin B and vitamin E, manganese, and fiber.

Clove's combination of vitamins and minerals is a great enhancement to chai tea. Clove is used to inhibit symptoms of gastrointestinal distress like constipation, diarrhea, and stomach cramps, and its aroma is known to reduce anxiety and stress.

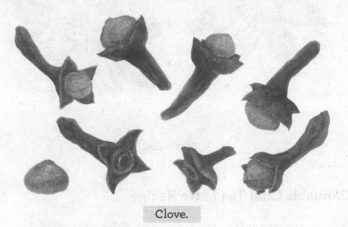

Clove.

Health Benefits of Star Anise

Star anise is made from the ground seeds of *Illicium verum*, a tree native to China whose seeds are encased within star-shaped pods. The spice contains bioactive compounds that provide antimicrobial, antioxidant, and anti-inflammatory properties. Star anise has been known to relieve inflammation, fight common flu symptoms, treat fungal infections, improve overall gut health, and promote sleep. Star anise has a great calming and soothing effect on the human mind and body.

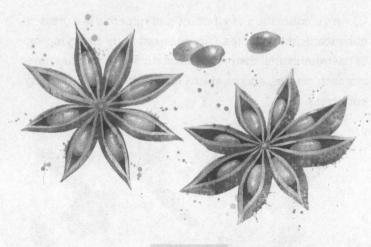

Star anise.

Cannabis Chai Tea Latte Recipe

Here is one of my favorite recipes to make a wonderful cannabis infused chai tea latte packed with powerful healing herbs and spices. This recipe will yield 24 ounces, so you will be able to save some to cool and reheat later. This recipe is just as delicious without the cannabis in it, but feel free to explore!

Tools Needed

- Medium saucepan
- Stove top or sous vide machine to warm water
- Small frying pan to toast herbs and spices (cast iron preferred)

Ingredients

- 2 cans full fat coconut milk
- 15 cardamom pods
- 8 whole black peppercorns
- 1 cinnamon stick
- 6 cloves
- 2 allspice berries
- 1 star of dry star anise
- 2 tablespoons black tea (any kind you like)
- Brown sugar
- Vanilla bean (¼-inch piece vanilla bean or ⅛ teaspoon vanilla extract)
- 1-inch piece of fresh ginger
- Cannabis flower (no need to decarb) or cannabis infusion

Instructions

1. Preheat a water bath to 185 degrees Fahrenheit, heating the water either on a stove top or using a sous vide machine. Make sure your water bath is the right size to fully cover a one-quart mason jar.
2. In a small frying pan over medium heat, toast the cardamom pods for 3 to 4 minutes, constantly moving the pan and stirring to make sure to prevent burning.
3. Add the whole black peppercorns to the pan and toast them with the cardamom pods for 3 to 4 minutes. Continue moving and stirring the contents of the pan to avoid burning.
4. Add the cinnamon stick, whole star anise, cloves, and allspice berries, and cook for 2 to 3 minutes. Your spices should be very fragrant with a light brown hue.

5. Shake coconut milk well in the mason jar and add in the brown sugar, black tea, cannabis flower or cannabis infusion, vanilla bean or extract, and fresh peeled ginger.
6. Once the spices are cool enough to safely touch, break the cinnamon stick down and crack open the cardamom pods by hand.
7. Add all of your spices to the coconut milk mixture in the mason jar and gently stir in.
8. Clean the edge of the mason jar with a cloth or paper towel, then place the lid on the jar, closing to finger tight (not all the way, just tight enough).
9. Lower the sealed mason jar into the water bath at 185 degrees and set a timer for 2 hours. Allow the mixture to cook undisturbed.
10. After 2 hours, carefully remove the mason jar and place it on top of a towel on the counter. Open the lid and gently stir.
11. Using a mesh strainer, a double layer of cheesecloth, or coffee filters, strain the tea into another mason jar or heat resistant container.
12. Enjoy your tea immediately or store for up to one week in the fridge!

Cannabis Canapés and Small Bites

I love appetizers! They are always my favorite thing on the menu, so what better way to start your cannabis culinary adventure off than with some canapés and small bites!

When we contemplate cannabis infused food, we often think about brownies and cookies. I do love to bake, and applying the infused cannabis butter recipe from earlier in the book to any of your favorite baking recipes will certainly upgrade any of your baked goods. But cannabis is an amazing ingredient with so much depth and complexity to explore that it should not be pigeonholed just into baking.

We will learn how to take some very basic infused oils and fats and turn them into kitchen staples that can be applied in many different directions and upgraded with tons of flavor combinations.

Here are some of my favorite things to serve at my house!

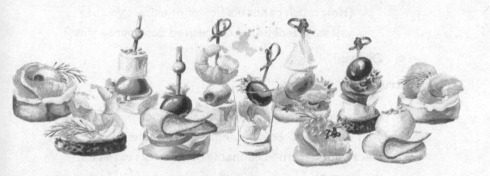

Canapés.

Cannabis Infused Olive Oil

Cannabis infused olive oil may be the most versatile ingredient in any cannabis culinary arsenal, bar none. Olive oil is highlighted in so many recipes. From simply dipping bread in balsamic vinegar and olive oil to using the oil as the base of mayonnaise, we see how far olive oil's influence truly extends in our kitchens.

We have already touched on a basic cannabis infusion in this chapter, but I will quickly recap how to make this culinary staple.

Tools Needed

- Stove or crock pot
- Small saucepan
- Whisk

Ingredients

- Decarboxylated cannabis or cannabis extract
  - ✦ (How much cannabis flower or extract you use will vary depending on desired dose per serving)
- Olive oil

Instructions

1. Using a sauce pan on the stove or a crock pot, warm your olive oil to 180–200 degrees Fahrenheit.
2. Place your decarbed cannabis or cannabis extract in the warm oil.
3. Leave on heat for 30 minutes, stirring occasionally.
4. Take off heat and let steep for another 30 minutes.
5. Strain through a mesh strainer and cheesecloth.

Your cannabis infused olive oil will last for six months in your pantry, and it may last even longer.

Roasted Beet Hummus

I love the color of beets but am not usually a fan of their intense earthy flavor. So when I first tried roasted beet hummus, I was slightly nervous. I was so wrong! It was absolutely delicious! The lemon, garlic, and olive oil temper the flavor of the beets perfectly.

The color of the dip is incredible! Essentially a shade of hot pink, it looks so beautiful in serving dishes, plus it's packed with chickpeas, a.k.a. garbanzo beans, a fantastic superfood full of protein, vitamins, and minerals.

This recipe is super simple once you have roasted your beets. All you need is a blender or food processor. It's also a great recipe because it keeps for about a week, providing a wonderful, healthy snack anytime!

Tools Needed

- ◆ Baking sheet
- ◆ Tin foil
- ◆ Blender or food processor
- ◆ Knife

Ingredients

- 1 small roasted beet
- 1 can of cooked chickpeas (90 percent drained)
- 1 large lemon, zested
- ½ large lemon, juiced
- 2 large cloves garlic, minced
- 2 heaping tablespoons tahini
- ¼ cup olive oil
- Served with pita bread or your choice of veggies

Instructions

1. Preheat your oven to 375 degrees Fahrenheit. Remove the stem from the beet and scrub and rinse it clean. Drizzle the beet with olive oil, then wrap in tin foil and roast in the oven for one hour. Once tender, set in fridge to cool.
2. Once your beet is cool, peel it and cut it into quarters, then place it in your food processor. Blend until only small bits remain.
3. Add remaining ingredients *except for olive oil*. Blend until smooth.
4. Drizzle in olive oil toward the end as the hummus is mixing.
5. Taste and adjust seasonings as needed, adding more salt, lemon juice, or olive oil if needed. If the hummus is too thick, you can add a bit of water.
6. Serve and enjoy!

Herb-Infused Honey

Honey is an incredible natural sweetener packed with many beneficial nutrients! You can make a honey infusion with a variety of herbs, not only cannabis; these honey infusions are delicious and can be very healing.

Herb-infused honey is a great way to use sprigs of fresh thyme and rosemary left over from cooking dinner, preserve a handful of mint, or elevate the flavor of the honey with some edible flowers. It couldn't be easier to do!

You can use herb-infused honey for so many things, from sweetening beverages to using it to a sweeten when baking. You can even stir it into marinades or salad dressings, or my favorite: serve herb-infused honey with a cheese plate.

Some herbal honey infusions are used medicinally; sage and honey is one classic honey infusion used for relieving a sore throat, while chamomile honey promotes calm and relaxation. Single herb honeys are the easiest to create, but feel free to get creative and try formulating your own blends.

Some of my favorite herbs to infuse, either singly or in various combinations, are rosemary, sage, thyme, mint, lemon balm, lavender, chamomile, pine tips, and rose petals. You can also use spices like star anise, a vanilla bean, or cinnamon sticks.

Your honey should be a nice light, mild color for the best infusion. Try buying local honey and supporting local farmers.

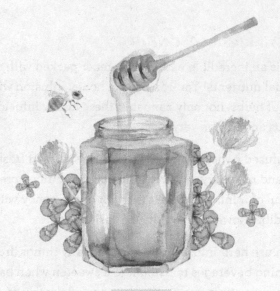

Honey.

To infuse honey with cannabis, try a cannabis extract or cannabis distillate. Cannabis distillates works great and are already decarboxylated. It has no flavor or smell, so it will not impact on your herbal infusion. Decarboxylated cannabis flower also works great.

Tools Needed

- ◆ Mason jars (pint or half pint)
- ◆ Chopstick or wooden handled spoon for stirring
- ◆ Clean cloth for wiping jar rims

Ingredients

- ◆ 1–2 tablespoons of dried herbs per 1 cup of honey
- ◆ Honey

Instructions for Preparing Cannabis Infusion:

1. Heat honey to a low simmer on a double boiler over medium heat, then reduce heat.
2. Mix in cannabis (extract or decarbed cannabis flower).
3. Let simmer for 20 minutes.
4. Take double boiler off heat.

Instructions:

1. Prepare your herbs in advance. All of the herbs for infusion should be dried. Herbs should be in the form of whole sprigs, buds, petals, or leaves; chopped herbs infuse faster but are harder to strain out. (To dry herbs, either leave them on your counter, on a baking sheet in the oven on low, or use your microwave.)
2. Place your herbs in the bottom of a jar, then fill the jar almost to the top with honey.
3. Using your stirring spoon or tool, stir in all of the herbs to be infused. Top up the jar and wipe the rim clean. Close jar lid tightly.
4. Let your herbs infuse into your honey for at least five days. If your herbs float to the top, flip the jar upside down, making sure the herbs are well-coated. For a more intense flavor, leave the herbs in for longer.
5. Strain the honey into a clean jar using a mesh strainer. If your honey is solid, pop it in the microwave for 10 to 20 seconds.
6. Store your honey in a tightly sealed jar in a cool dry place; it will last indefinitely!

Cannabis Infused Mayonnaise

Making your own mayo at home may seem intimidating at first, but once you realize how simple it is to make with ingredients you always have on hand, you'll wonder why you ever bought it in the first place. On top of that, homemade mayo is incredibly delicious and easy to customize.

Mayonnaise may be a sandwich staple but is also extremely versatile in the kitchen, with applications across many dishes. When you consider the simple ingredients that make up mayo—eggs and oil—it's no wonder that it is used to moisten so many recipes.

The days of no mayo should be behind us. When we get to choose the quality of our ingredients, the flavor profile is unlimited! As always, choose the best ingredients for your cooking, and why not try exploring different olive oils? Do you know of an olive oil store in your city? Try and find one. There are so many olive oils to explore, and fresher is always better!

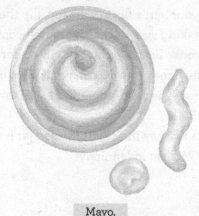

Mayo.

Tools Needed

◆ Food processor

Ingredients

◆ 1 egg
◆ ½ tablespoon lemon juice
◆ 1 teaspoon white wine vinegar
◆ ¼ teaspoon Dijon mustard
◆ ¼ teaspoon sea salt
◆ 1 cup of avocado oil or lightly flavored olive oil

Instructions

1. Add the egg to the bowl of the food processor and process for about 20 seconds.
2. Add the mustard salt, lemon, vinegar, and mustard and process again for 20 seconds.
3. *Slowly* add the oil in tiny drops as the food processor is processing. If you do not add it *very slowly,* you will have a broken mayonnaise soup.
4. Taste your mayo and season to taste with salt, vinegar, or lemon juice.
5. Classic mayo rocks by itself, but feel free to spice it up with other fresh herbs, roasted garlic, chipotle, curry powder, or sriracha sauce.

Parmesan Crostini

Parmesan crostini is the ultimate form of cheese on crackers! It's something so deliciously brilliant, nobody could turn it down. This easy appetizer is ready in five minutes (and will probably take half that time to devour).

The first time I saw this recipe was I believe on a box of Ritz crackers, so I knew it was going to be delicious. Use infused mayonnaise to upgrade this snack! Make sure the cannabis dose isn't too high because I guarantee you will want to eat more than a few.

To prepare your crostini, first cut thin rounds or cut points out of a baguette (or any bread you desire). Toast until nice and crispy to a crumble.

Tools Needed

- ◆ Baking sheet
- ◆ Tin foil
- ◆ Oven

Ingredients

- ◆ 1 cup of mayonnaise
- ◆ ¾ cup grated parmesan cheese
- ◆ ⅓ cup thinly sliced green onions
- ◆ 30 crostinis or crackers.

Instructions

1. Preheat broiler, briefly using the broil setting on the oven.
2. Mix mayo, parmesan cheese, and onions until well blended.
3. Spread onto crackers and place on foil lined baking sheet.
4. Place in oven and broil for 2 to 3 minutes, or until cheese and mayo mixture is golden brown.
5. Serve warm and enjoy!

Hot Swiss Cheese Dip

Here is a quick, simple, and delicious appetizer that will leave everyone asking for more! With equal amounts of all ingredients, this is a foolproof showstopper.

Your dip will be instantly upgraded by using the homemade mayonnaise we tried earlier. If you are reaching for store-bought mayo, at least look for those made from scratch from real ingredients, and try to avoid highly processed ingredients like soybean oil.

If you are allergic to eggs and would like to try this recipe without the mayo, try using whole milk Greek yogurt. It's not quite as good but still delicious.

Tools Needed

- ◆ Cutting board
- ◆ Cheese grater
- ◆ Knife
- ◆ Bowl
- ◆ Baking dish or ramekins

Ingredients

- ◆ 1 cup of mayonnaise
- ◆ 1 cup of shredded swiss cheese
- ◆ 1 cup of chopped sweet onion
- ◆ Served with toasted baguette or other bread slices or crackers

Instructions

1. Mix the onions, mayonnaise, and cheese in a bowl, then spoon into a one-quart baking dish, pie dish, or several small ramekins.
2. Bake at 350 degrees F for 25 to 30 minutes or until bubbly golden brown on top.
3. Remove from oven and serve with bread or crackers.
4. Enjoy!

Bruschetta

Bruschetta is a deliciously classic way to enjoy simple, fresh ingredients. Pronounced "brusketta," this Italian classic perfectly captures all of the flavors of garden ripe tomatoes, fresh basil, garlic, and olive oil.

My mom taught me how to make bruschetta, and it couldn't be any easier; it's just a mixture of a few simple chopped ingredients, spooned over slices of toasted baguette or rustic bread brushed with olive oil.

It's a perfect party food because you can make a large batch of it ahead of time and it lasts for up to a week in your fridge. Make sure to toast extra pieces of bread! You'll always want more.

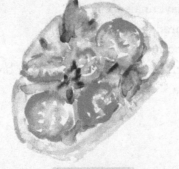

Bruschetta.

This is a pretty big batch, so feel free to cut it in half if you are not feeding a family of four or planning on making enough for extras.

Tools Needed

- Knife
- Cutting board
- Bowl
- Served with: olive oil brushed toasted bread (French baguette or similar)

Ingredients

- 6 or 7 ripe tomatoes (1½ pounds)
- 2 cloves garlic, minced (or 2 heaping teaspoons)
- 1 tablespoon extra virgin olive oil
- 1 teaspoon balsamic vinegar
- 6 to 8 large fresh basil leaves, finely sliced or chopped
- ¾ teaspoon sea salt
- ½ teaspoon freshly ground pepper
- ¼ cup of olive oil

Instructions

1. Chop your tomatoes down to small pieces.
2. In a bowl, combine all of your ingredients and toss.
3. Serve on toasted bread slices and enjoy!

The Future
of Cannabis

Cannabis is becoming rapidly normalized in our society.
What once was a fringe drug is now seen as a real therapeutic
medicine as well as a low-risk intoxicant. Cannabis has so
many medical benefits; the list seems endless. We have many
well researched studies on everything from how cannabis
can attack specific cancer cells, stopping them in their tracks,
to how it helps people manage everyday pain and anxiety.
Cannabis is much more than just a drug; it is a plant that
you can grow at home. It is a natural and holistic medicine
that can easily be cultivated and obtained in most areas. The
United Nations recently reclassified cannabis from being a
dangerous drug to classifying it as a plant with medicinal
value. This ruling shows the global reach that cannabis is
having today.

With many places all over the world legalizing cannabis for
recreational use, its value beyond the medicinal is immense.
Cannabis is a far-reaching industry with a multi-billion-dollar
market cap that is nowhere close to being met. Canada has
had cannabis legalization since October 17, 2018, and has
seen immense tax profits and job creation from legalization.
We have seen a wide and sweeping acceptance of cannabis
use, and its normalization has been expedited by consumer

acceptance. Canada may be one of the first, but it will not soon be the last.

In the coming years, we will see a tidal wave of cannabis legalization. As you read this, cannabis may recently have been legalized where you live. In the last few years, we have been seeing cannabis legalization efforts charging forward, with Mexico's vote to legalize cannabis before the end of 2020 and the Marijuana Opportunity, Reinvestment, and Expungement (MORE) Act's passage by the House of Representatives in the United States. The handwriting is on the wall that we will soon see cannabis prohibition come to an end.

Whether you use cannabis as a medicine, intoxicant, relaxant, social connection enhancer, or all of the above, we will soon see cannabis destigmatized in the eyes of our peers. Cannabis has the opportunity to help connect the world and heal some of the damage that has been done by the failed war on drugs.

Congratulations, drugs, you won the war on drugs.

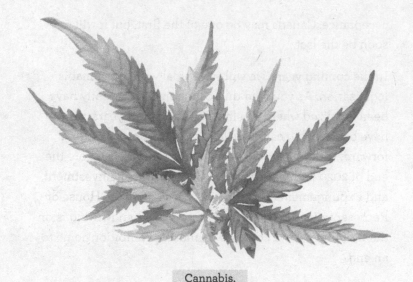

Cannabis.

A Final Word on Terpenes

The world of scent is vast and deep, complex and arousing. Our sense of smell is constantly bombarded with the delicious, the fragrant, the weird, and sometimes the awkward.

Throughout this book, we have learned to identify, categorize, and appreciate different aromas for their distinct impacts on human's physical and metaphysical well-being.

Together, we have dived into our sense of smell more deeply than we thought possible and have learned to harness common scents to benefit our well-being.

We are surrounded by natural healing powers that can be unlocked as long as we look deep enough.

Resources

Acne.org. "Jojoba Oil." Accessed February 5, 2021. https://www.acne.org/jojoba-oil.html.

Akilen, Rajadurai, Zeller Pimlott, Amalia Tsiami, and Nicola Robinson. "Effect of Short-Term Administration of Cinnamon on Blood Pressure in Patients with Prediabetes and Type 2 Diabetes." *Nutrition (Burbank, Los Angeles County, Calif.)* 29, no. 10 (October 2013): 1192–96. https://doi.org/10.1016/j.nut.2013.03.007.

Ali, Babar, Naser Ali Al-Wabel, Saiba Shams, Aftab Ahamad, Shah Alam Khan, and Firoz Anwar. "Essential Oils Used in Aromatherapy: A Systemic Review." *Asian Pacific Journal of Tropical Biomedicine* 5, no. 8 (August 1, 2015): 601–11. https://doi.org/10.1016/j.apjtb.2015.05.007.

American College of Healthcare Sciences. "3 Common and Dangerous Essential Oil Mistakes | Achs.Edu." Accessed February 5, 2021. https://info.achs.edu/blog/aromatherapy-essential-oil-dangers-and-safety.

Amsterdam, Jay D., Yimei Li, Irene Soeller, Kenneth Rockwell, Jun James Mao, and Justine Shults. "A Randomized, Double-Blind, Placebo-Controlled Trial of Oral Matricaria Recutita (Chamomile) Extract Therapy for Generalized Anxiety Disorder." *Journal of Clinical Psychopharmacology* 29, no. 4 (August 2009): 378–82. https://doi.org/10.1097/JCP.0b013e3181ac935c.

Aurora Health Care. "Aromatherapy: The Art and Science of Using Essential Oils." (2018): www.aurorahealthcare.

org/~/media/aurorahealthcareorg/documents/integra-
tive-medicine/aromatherapy-essential-oils.pdf.

Ben Hsouna, Anis, Nihed Ben Halima, Slim Smaoui, and Naceur
Hamdi. "Citrus Lemon Essential Oil: Chemical Composition, Antioxidant and Antimicrobial Activities with
Its Preservative Effect against Listeria Monocytogenes
Inoculated in Minced Beef Meat." *Lipids in Health
and Disease* 16, no. 1 (August 3, 2017): 146. https://doi.
org/10.1186/s12944-017-0487-5.

Booth, Judith K., Jonathan E. Page, and Jörg Bohlmann. "Terpene Synthases from Cannabis Sativa." *PLoS ONE* 12,
no. 3 (March 29, 2017). https://doi.org/10.1371/journal.
pone.0173911.

Burcu, Gul Baykalir, Ciftci Osman, Cetin Aslı, Oztanir Mustafa
Namik, Basak Türkmen Neşe, Gul Baykalir Burcu, Ciftci
Osman, Cetin Aslı, Oztanir Mustafa Namik, and Basak
Türkmen Neşe. "The Protective Cardiac Effects of
B-Myrcene after Global Cerebral Ischemia/Reperfusion
in C57BL/J6 Mouse." *Acta Cirúrgica Brasileira* 31, no.
7 (July 2016): 456–62. https://doi.org/10.1590/S0102-
865020160070000005.

Burns, E., C. Blamey, S. J. Ersser, A. J. Lloyd, and L. Barnetson.
"The Use of Aromatherapy in Intrapartum Midwifery
Practice an Observational Study." *Complementary Therapies in Nursing & Midwifery* 6, no. 1 (February 2000):
33–34. https://doi.org/10.1054/ctnm.1999.0901.

Cássia da Silveira e Sá, Rita de, Tamires Cardoso Lima, Flávio
Rogério da Nóbrega, Anna Emmanuela Medeiros
de Brito, and Damião Pergentino de Sousa. "Analge-
sic-Like Activity of Essential Oil Constituents: An
Update." *International Journal of Molecular Sciences*

18, no. 12 (December 9, 2017). https://doi.org/10.3390/ijms18122392.

Cavanagh, H. M. A., and J. M. Wilkinson. "Biological Activities of Lavender Essential Oil." *Phytotherapy Research* 16, no. 4 (2002): 301–8. https://doi.org/10.1002/ptr.1103.

"CFR - Code of Federal Regulations Title 21." Accessed February 5, 2021. https://www.accessdata.fda.gov/scripts/cdrh/cfdocs/cfcfr/CFRSearch.cfm?fr=182.20.

Chang, So Young. "Effects of aroma hand massage on pain, state anxiety and depression in hospice patients with terminal cancer." *Taehan Kanho Hakhoe Chi* 38, no. 4 (August 2008): 493–502. https://doi.org/10.4040/jkan.2008.38.4.493.

Chen, Jun, Qiu-Dong Jiang, Ya-Ping Chai, Hui Zhang, Pei Peng, and Xi-Xiong Yang. "Natural Terpenes as Penetration Enhancers for Transdermal Drug Delivery." *Molecules* 21, no. 12 (December 11, 2016). https://doi.org/10.3390/molecules21121709.

Chin, Karen B., and Barbara Cordell. "The Effect of Tea Tree Oil (Melaleuca Alternifolia) on Wound Healing Using a Dressing Model." *The Journal of Alternative and Complementary Medicine* 19, no. 12 (July 13, 2013): 942–45. https://doi.org/10.1089/acm.2012.0787.

Cho, Kyoung Sang, Young-ran Lim, Kyungho Lee, Jaeseok Lee, Jang Ho Lee, and Im-Soon Lee. "Terpenes from Forests and Human Health." *Toxicological Research* 33, no. 2 (April 2017): 97–106. https://doi.org/10.5487/TR.2017.33.2.097.

Chouhan, Sonam, Kanika Sharma, and Sanjay Guleria. "Antimicrobial Activity of Some Essential Oils—Present Status and Future Perspectives." *Medicines* 4, no. 3 (August 8,

2017). https://doi.org/10.3390/medicines4030058.

Cohen, Marc Maurice. "Tulsi - Ocimum Sanctum: A Herb for All Reasons." *Journal of Ayurveda and Integrative Medicine* 5, no. 4 (2014): 251–59. https://doi.org/10.4103/0975-9476.146554.

Cox-Georgian, Destinney, Niveditha Ramadoss, Chathu Dona, and Chhandak Basu. "Therapeutic and Medicinal Uses of Terpenes." *Medicinal Plants*, November 12, 2019, 333–59. https://doi.org/10.1007/978-3-030-31269-5_15.

Encyclopedia Britannica. "Isoprenoid | Chemical Compound." Accessed February 5, 2021. https://www.britannica.com/science/isoprenoid.

"Essential Oils: Poisonous When Misused." Accessed February 5, 2021. https://www.poison.org/articles/2014-jun/essential-oils.

Federation of Holistic Therapists Directory Service. "Aromatherapy." Accessed February 5, 2021. https://www.fht.org.uk/therapies/aromatherapy.

Frass, Michael, Robert Paul Strassl, Helmut Friehs, Michael Müllner, Michael Kundi, and Alan D. Kaye. "Use and Acceptance of Complementary and Alternative Medicine Among the General Population and Medical Personnel: A Systematic Review." *The Ochsner Journal* 12, no. 1 (2012): 45–56.

Freeman, Jennifer. "RA Essential Oils: What Essential Oils Are Anti-Inflammatory? - RheumatoidArthritis.Org." https://www.rheumatoidarthritis.org/. Accessed February 5, 2021. https://www.rheumatoidarthritis.org/living-with-ra/diet/essential-oils/.

Funk, Janet L., Jennifer B. Frye, Janice N. Oyarzo, Huaping Zhang, and Barbara N. Timmermann. "Anti-Arthritic

Effects and Toxicity of the Essential Oils of Turmeric (Curcuma Longa L.)." *Journal of Agricultural and Food Chemistry* 58, no. 2 (January 27, 2010): 842–49. https://doi.org/10.1021/jf9027206.

Gnatta, Juliana Rizzo, Patricia Petrone Piason, Cristiane de Lion Botero Couto Lopes, Noemi Marisa Brunet Rogenski, and Maria Júlia Paes da Silva. "Aromatherapy with ylang ylang for anxiety and self-esteem: a pilot study." *Revista Da Escola De Enfermagem Da U S P* 48, no. 3 (June 2014): 492–99. https://doi.org/10.1590/s0080-623420140000300015.

Goel, Namni, Hyungsoo Kim, and Raymund P. Lao. "An Olfactory Stimulus Modifies Nighttime Sleep in Young Men and Women." *Chronobiology International* 22, no. 5 (January 1, 2005): 889–904. https://doi.org/10.1080/07420520500263276.

Goes, Tiago Costa, Fabrício Dias Antunes, Péricles Barreto Alves, and Flavia Teixeira-Silva. "Effect of Sweet Orange Aroma on Experimental Anxiety in Humans." *Journal of Alternative and Complementary Medicine (New York, N.Y.)* 18, no. 8 (August 2012): 798–804. https://doi.org/10.1089/acm.2011.0551.

Hamidpour, Rafie, Soheila Hamidpour, Mohsen Hamidpour, and Mina Shahlari. "Camphor (Cinnamomum Camphora), a Traditional Remedy with the History of Treating Several Diseases." *International Journal of Case Reports and Images (IJCRI)* 4, no. 2 (October 24, 2013): 86–89. https://doi.org/10.5348/ijcri-2013-02-267-RA-1.

Han, Fei, Guang-qiang Ma, Ming Yang, Li Yan, Wei Xiong, Ji-cheng Shu, Zhi-dong Zhao, and Han-lin Xu. "Chemical Composition and Antioxidant Activities of Essential

Oils from Different Parts of the Oregano." *Journal of Zhejiang University. Science. B* 18, no. 1 (January 2017): 79–84. https://doi.org/10.1631/jzus.B1600377.

Han, Xuesheng, Damian Rodriguez, and Tory L. Parker. "Biological Activities of Frankincense Essential Oil in Human Dermal Fibroblasts." *Biochimie Open* 4 (June 1, 2017): 31–35. https://doi.org/10.1016/j.biopen.2017.01.003.

Health Canada. "Cannabis Market Data." Datasets. aem, September 18, 2020. https://www.canada.ca/en/health-canada/services/drugs-medication/cannabis/research-data/market.html.

Heggers, John P., John Cottingham, Jean Gusman, Lana Reagor, Lana McCoy, Edith Carino, Robert Cox, and Jian-Gang Zhao. "The Effectiveness of Processed Grapefruit-Seed Extract as An Antibacterial Agent: II. Mechanism of Action and In Vitro Toxicity." *The Journal of Alternative and Complementary Medicine* 8, no. 3 (June 1, 2002): 333–40. https://doi.org/10.1089/10755530260128023.

Herbal Academy. "The Truth About Phototoxic Essential Oils & How To Use Them Safely," July 11, 2016. https://theherbalacademy.com/truth-phototoxic-essential-oils-use-safely/.

Herbal Academy. "Using Essential Oils for Children - Herbal Academy of New England," August 15, 2014. https://theherbalacademy.com/using-essential-oils-for-children/.

Hongratanaworakit, Tapanee, and Gerhard Buchbauer. "Relaxing Effect of Ylang Ylang Oil on Humans after Transdermal Absorption." *Phytotherapy Research* 20, no. 9 (2006): 758–63. https://doi.org/10.1002/ptr.1950.

Hur, Myung-Haeng, Ji-Ah Song, Jeonghee Lee, and Myeong Soo Lee. "Aromatherapy for Stress Reduction in Healthy

Adults: A Systematic Review and Meta-Analysis of Randomized Clinical Trials." *Maturitas* 79, no. 4 (December 2014): 362–69. https://doi.org/10.1016/j.maturitas.2014.08.006.

Jun, Yang Suk, Purum Kang, Sun Seek Min, Jeong-Min Lee, Hyo-Keun Kim, and Geun Hee Seol. "Effect of Eucalyptus Oil Inhalation on Pain and Inflammatory Responses after Total Knee Replacement: A Randomized Clinical Trial." *Evidence-Based Complementary and Alternative Medicine* 2013 (2013).

Klauke, A.-L., I. Racz, B. Pradier, A. Markert, A. M. Zimmer, J. Gertsch, and A. Zimmer. "The Cannabinoid CB₂ Receptor-Selective Phytocannabinoid Beta-Caryophyllene Exerts Analgesic Effects in Mouse Models of Inflammatory and Neuropathic Pain." *European Neuropsychopharmacology: The Journal of the European College of Neuropsychopharmacology* 24, no. 4 (April 2014): 608–20. https://doi.org/10.1016/j.euroneuro.2013.10.008.

Lafaye, Genevieve, Laurent Karila, Lisa Blecha, and Amine Benyamina. "Cannabis, Cannabinoids, and Health." *Dialogues in Clinical Neuroscience* 19, no. 3 (September 2017): 309–16.

Linus Pauling Institute. "Vitamin C and Skin Health," November 7, 2016. https://lpi.oregonstate.edu/mic/health-disease/skin-health/vitamin-C.

Man, Adrian, Luigi Santacroce, Romeo Iacob, Anca Mare, and Lidia Man. "Antimicrobial Activity of Six Essential Oils Against a Group of Human Pathogens: A Comparative Study." *Pathogens* 8, no. 1 (March 2019): 15. https://doi.org/10.3390/pathogens8010015.

Marzouk, Tyseer MF, Amina MR El-Nemer, and Hany N. Baraka.

"The Effect of Aromatherapy Abdominal Massage on Alleviating Menstrual Pain in Nursing Students: A Prospective Randomized Cross-over Study." *Evidence-Based Complementary and Alternative Medicine* 2013 (2013).

Meamarbashi, Abbas. "Instant Effects of Peppermint Essential Oil on the Physiological Parameters and Exercise Performance." *Avicenna Journal of Phytomedicine* 4, no. 1 (2014): 72–78.

Mohammadhosseini, Majid, Satyajit D. Sarker, and Abolfazl Akbarzadeh. "Chemical Composition of the Essential Oils and Extracts of Achillea Species and Their Biological Activities: A Review." *Journal of Ethnopharmacology* 199 (March 6, 2017): 257–315. https://doi.org/10.1016/j.jep.2017.02.010.

Mohebitabar, Safieh, Mahboobeh Shirazi, Sodabeh Bioos, Roja Rahimi, Farhad Malekshahi, and Fatemeh Nejatbakhsh. "Therapeutic Efficacy of Rose Oil: A Comprehensive Review of Clinical Evidence." *Avicenna Journal of Phytomedicine* 7, no. 3 (2017): 206–13.

Morales, Paula, Dow P. Hurst, and Patricia H. Reggio. "Molecular Targets of the Phytocannabinoids-A Complex Picture." *Progress in the Chemistry of Organic Natural Products* 103 (2017): 103–31. https://doi.org/10.1007/978-3-319-45541-9_4.

Mori, Hiroko-Miyuki, Hiroshi Kawanami, Hirohisa Kawahata, and Motokuni Aoki. "Wound Healing Potential of Lavender Oil by Acceleration of Granulation and Wound Contraction through Induction of TGF-β in a Rat Model." *BMC Complementary and Alternative Medicine* 16, no. 1 (May 26, 2016): 144. https://doi.org/10.1186/s12906-

016-1128-7.

"Most Commonly Used Essential Oils | National Association for Holistic Aromatherapy." Accessed February 5, 2021. https://naha.org/index.php/explore-aromatherapy/about-aromatherapy/most-commonly-used-essential-oils.

Nagatomo, Akifumi, Norihisa Nishida, Ikuo Fukuhara, Akira Noro, Yoshimichi Kozai, Hisao Sato, and Yoichi Matsuura. "Daily Intake of Rosehip Extract Decreases Abdominal Visceral Fat in Preobese Subjects: A Randomized, Double-Blind, Placebo-Controlled Clinical Trial." *Diabetes, Metabolic Syndrome and Obesity: Targets and Therapy* 8 (March 6, 2015): 147–56. https://doi.org/10.2147/DMSO.S78623.

"NAHA | Exploring Aromatherapy." Accessed February 5, 2021. https://naha.org/index.php/explore-aromatherapy/safety.

"NAHA | Exploring Aromatherapy." Accessed February 5, 2021. https://naha.org/index.php/explore-aromatherapy/about-aromatherapy/methods-of-application.

National Institute on Drug Abuse. "What Is the Scope of Marijuana Use in the United States?" National Institute on Drug Abuse, --. https://www.drugabuse.gov/publications/research-reports/marijuana/what-scope-marijuana-use-in-united-states.

Nazaruk, J., and M. Borzym-Kluczyk. "The Role of Triterpenes in the Management of Diabetes Mellitus and Its Complications." *Phytochemistry Reviews* 14, no. 4 (2015): 675–90. https://doi.org/10.1007/s11101-014-9369-x.

NCCIH. "Peppermint Oil." Accessed February 5, 2021. https://www.nccih.nih.gov/health/peppermint-oil.

NCCIH. "Sage." Accessed February 5, 2021. https://www.nccih. nih.gov/health/sage.

NCCIH. "Tea Tree Oil." Accessed February 5, 2021. https://www. nccih.nih.gov/health/tea-tree-oil.

NHS. "Cannabis: The Facts," April 26, 2018. https://www.nhs.uk/ live-well/healthy-body/cannabis-the-facts/.

Nosrati, Simin, S. A. Esmailzadeh-Hosseini, Abolfzl Sarpeleh, Mahmoud Soflaei Shahrbabak, and Yeganeh Soflaei Shahrbabak. "Antifungal Activity of Spearmint (Mentha Spicata L.) Essential Oil on Fusarium Oxysporum f. Sp. Radiciscucumerinum the Causal Agent of Stem and Crown Rot of Greenhouse Cucumber in Yazd, Iran." In *International Conference on Environmental and Agricultural Engineering, Chengdu, China Held On,* 2011:52–56, 2011.

Oakley, Amanda, Vanessa Ngan, and Clare Morrison. "What Causes Acne?" DermNet. (2014). www.dermnetnz.org/ topics/what-causes-acne.

Oboh, Ganiyu, Ifeoluwa A. Akinbola, Ayokunle O. Ademosun, David M. Sanni, Oluwatoyin V. Odubanjo, Tosin A. Olasehinde, and Sunday I. Oyeleye. "Essential Oil from Clove Bud (*Eugenia Aromatica* Kuntze) Inhibit Key Enzymes Relevant to the Management of Type-2 Diabetes and Some Pro-Oxidant Induced Lipid Peroxidation in Rats Pancreas *in Vitro.*" *Journal of Oleo Science* 64, no. 7 (2015): 775–82. https://doi.org/10.5650/jos.ess14274.

Orchard, Ané, and Sandy van Vuuren. "Commercial Essential Oils as Potential Antimicrobials to Treat Skin Diseases." *Evidence-Based Complementary and Alternative Medicine: ECAM* 2017 (2017). https://doi. org/10.1155/2017/4517971.

Ou, Ming-Chiu, Yu-Fei Lee, Chih-Ching Li, and Shyi-Kuen Wu. "The Effectiveness of Essential Oils for Patients with Neck Pain: A Randomized Controlled Study." *The Journal of Alternative and Complementary Medicine* 20, no. 10 (September 5, 2014): 771–79. https://doi.org/10.1089/acm.2013.0453.

Pamplona, Fabricio A., Lorenzo Rolim da Silva, and Ana Carolina Coan. "Potential Clinical Benefits of CBD-Rich Cannabis Extracts Over Purified CBD in Treatment-Resistant Epilepsy: Observational Data Meta-Analysis." *Frontiers in Neurology* 9 (September 12, 2018). https://doi.org/10.3389/fneur.2018.00759.

Pazyar, Nader, Reza Yaghoobi, Nooshin Bagherani, and Afshin Kazerouni. "A Review of Applications of Tea Tree Oil in Dermatology." *International Journal of Dermatology* 52, no. 7 (2013): 784–90. https://doi.org/10.1111/j.1365-4632.2012.05654.x.

Pereira, Effie J, Lauren Sim, Helen S Driver, Chris M Parker, and Michael F Fitzpatrick. "The Effect of Inhaled Menthol on Upper Airway Resistance in Humans: A Randomized Controlled Crossover Study." *Canadian Respiratory Journal : Journal of the Canadian Thoracic Society* 20, no. 1 (2013): e1–4.

Pereira, Irina, Patrícia Severino, Ana C. Santos, Amélia M. Silva, and Eliana B. Souto. "Linalool Bioactive Properties and Potential Applicability in Drug Delivery Systems." *Colloids and Surfaces B: Biointerfaces* 171 (November 1, 2018): 566–78. https://doi.org/10.1016/j.colsurfb.2018.08.001.

Rao, Pasupuleti Visweswara, and Siew Hua Gan. "Cinnamon: A Multifaceted Medicinal Plant." *Evidence-Based Comple-*

mentary and Alternative Medicine 2014 (2014).

Russo, Ethan B. "The Case for the Entourage Effect and Conventional Breeding of Clinical Cannabis: No 'Strain,' No Gain." *Frontiers in Plant Science* 9 (January 9, 2019). https://doi.org/10.3389/fpls.2018.01969.

Santiago, Marina, Shivani Sachdev, Jonathon C. Arnold, Iain S. McGregor, and Mark Connor. "Absence of Entourage: Terpenoids Commonly Found in Cannabis Sativa Do Not Modulate the Functional Activity of Δ9-THC at Human CB1 and CB2 Receptors." *Cannabis and Cannabinoid Research* 4, no. 3 (July 29, 2019): 165–76. https://doi.org/10.1089/can.2019.0016.

Sasannejad, Payam, Morteza Saeedi, Ali Shoeibi, Ali Gorji, Maryam Abbasi, and Mohsen Foroughipour. "Lavender Essential Oil in the Treatment of Migraine Headache: A Placebo-Controlled Clinical Trial." *European Neurology* 67, no. 5 (2012): 288–91. https://doi.org/10.1159/000335249.

Schnitzler, P., K. Schön, and J. Reichling. "Antiviral Activity of Australian Tea Tree Oil and Eucalyptus Oil against Herpes Simplex Virus in Cell Culture." *Die Pharmazie* 56, no. 4 (April 2001): 343–47.

ScienceDirect. "Monoterpenoid." (2019) Accessed February 5, 2021. https://www.sciencedirect.com/topics/medicine-and-dentistry/monoterpenoid.

Sharifi-Rad, Javad, Antoni Sureda, Gian Carlo Tenore, Maria Daglia, Mehdi Sharifi-Rad, Marco Valussi, Rosa Tundis, et al. "Biological Activities of Essential Oils: From Plant Chemoecology to Traditional Healing Systems." *Molecules : A Journal of Synthetic Chemistry and Natural Product Chemistry* 22, no. 1 (January 1, 2017). https://doi.

org/10.3390/molecules22010070.

Sharma, M., C. Levenson, R. H. Bell, S. A. Anderson, J. B. Hudson, C. C. Collins, and M. E. Cox. "Suppression of Lipopolysaccharide-Stimulated Cytokine/Chemokine Production in Skin Cells by Sandalwood Oils and Purified α-Santalol and β-Santalol." *Phytotherapy Research* 28, no. 6 (2014): 925–32. https://doi.org/10.1002/ptr.5080.

Sieniawska, Elwira, Rafal Sawicki, Marta Swatko-Ossor, Agnieszka Napiorkowska, Agata Przekora, Grazyna Ginalska, and Ewa Augustynowicz-Kopec. "The Effect of Combining Natural Terpenes and Antituberculous Agents against Reference and Clinical Mycobacterium Tuberculosis Strains." *Molecules : A Journal of Synthetic Chemistry and Natural Product Chemistry* 23, no. 1 (January 15, 2018). https://doi.org/10.3390/molecules23010176.

Silva, Joyce Kelly R. da, Pablo Luis Baia Figueiredo, Kendall G. Byler, and William N. Setzer. "Essential Oils as Antiviral Agents, Potential of Essential Oils to Treat SARS-CoV-2 Infection: An In-Silico Investigation." *International Journal of Molecular Sciences* 21, no. 10 (May 12, 2020). https://doi.org/10.3390/ijms21103426.

Sousa, Damião Pergentino de, Palloma de Almeida Soares Hocayen, Luciana Nalone Andrade, and Roberto Andreatini. "A Systematic Review of the Anxiolytic-Like Effects of Essential Oils in Animal Models." *Molecules* 20, no. 10 (October 14, 2015): 18620–60. https://doi.org/10.3390/molecules201018620.

Srivastava, Janmejai K., Eswar Shankar, and Sanjay Gupta. "Chamomile: A Herbal Medicine of the Past with a Bright Future (Review)." *Molecular Medicine Reports*

3, no. 6 (November 1, 2010): 895–901. https://doi.
org/10.3892/mmr.2010.377.

Stea, Susanna, Alina Beraudi, and Dalila De Pasquale. "Essential
Oils for Complementary Treatment of Surgical Patients:
State of the Art." *Evidence-Based Complementary and
Alternative Medicine* 2014 (2014).

Tan, Ji Wei, Daud Ahmad Israf, and Chau Ling Tham. "Major
Bioactive Compounds in Essential Oils Extracted
From the Rhizomes of Zingiber Zerumbet (L) Smith: A
Mini-Review on the Anti-Allergic and Immunomodula-
tory Properties." *Frontiers in Pharmacology* 9 (June 20,
2018). https://doi.org/10.3389/fphar.2018.00652.

Tisser, Hana. "Bath Safety." Tisserand Institute. Accessed February 5, 2021. https://tisserandinstitute.org/learn-more/
bath-safety-2/.

The School of Aromatic Studies. "Undiluted Application of Essential Oils," February 3, 2013. https://aromaticstudies.
com/undiluted-application-of-essential-oils/.

"Vegetable Oil | Cosmetics Info." Accessed February 5, 2021.
https://cosmeticsinfo.org/ingredient/vegetable-oil.

Vieira, A. J., F. P. Beserra, M. C. Souza, B. M. Totti, and A. L.
Rozza. "Limonene: Aroma of Innovation in Health and
Disease." *Chemico-Biological Interactions* 283 (March 1,
2018): 97–106. https://doi.org/10.1016/j.cbi.2018.02.007.

Weston-Green, Katrina. "The United Chemicals of Cannabis:
Beneficial Effects of Cannabis Phytochemicals on the
Brain and Cognition." *Recent Advances in Cannabinoid
Research*, November 5, 2018. https://doi.org/10.5772/
intechopen.79266.

Wu, Shuhua, Krupa B Patel, Leland J Booth, Jordan P Metcalf,
Hsueh-Kung Lin, and Wenxin Wu. "Protective Essential

Oil Attenuates Influenza Virus Infection: An in Vitro Study in MDCK Cells." *BMC Complementary and Alternative Medicine* 10 (November 15, 2010): 69. https://doi.org/10.1186/1472-6882-10-69.

Yip, Yin Bing, and Ada Chung Ying Tam. "An Experimental Study on the Effectiveness of Massage with Aromatic Ginger and Orange Essential Oil for Moderate-to-Severe Knee Pain among the Elderly in Hong Kong." *Complementary Therapies in Medicine* 16, no. 3 (June 1, 2008): 131–38. https://doi.org/10.1016/j.ctim.2007.12.003.

Acknowledgements

This book is dedicated to everyone who fought the ridiculous and ludicrous war on drugs. Thank you for standing up for what is right and allowing people to have the access to a plant that they deserve!

I'd like to thank the amazing people at Mango Publishing for believing in my ideas! Thank you kindly to my editor, Yaddyra Peralta. Thank you, Lisa McGuinness for finding me and setting this whole process in motion. Thank you to my wonderful wife Sarah for believing in me and my ideas. Thank you for letting me believe in me. Thank you to my mom Diana for loving aromatherapy and always buying me cool essential oils and teaching me about holistic medicine. Thank you to my dad Michael for reading my ramblings. Thank you to everyone who ever wrote a book, it's not easy!

Thank you to Gary Vaynerchuk, the best mentor I never had; I hope I can send you a copy of this book and tell you how much your inspiration meant to my journey. A huge shout-out to everyone pushing the cannabis culinary world forward, including Chef Manny Mendoza, Chef Nate Santana, Chef Jordan Wagman, Javier Garcia (Big Mich), Chef David Yusefzadeh, Ry Prichard, and so many more.

And finally, my thanks to you, the person reading this. Without you, there would be no book! I appreciate you so much!

About the Author

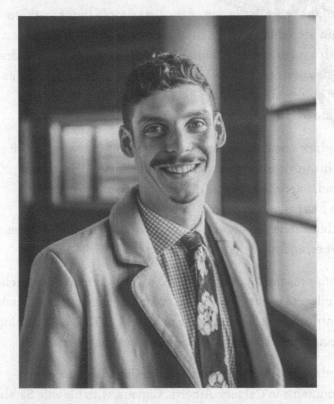

Andrew Freedman is "The Cannabis Sommelier," an international speaker, podcast host, YouTube personality, and now author!

Andrew saw a massive gap in the cannabis industry and knew he could change the dialogue around cannabis using the vernacular of fine wines. He dove down the rabbit hole of tasting terpenes and flavonoids and became obsessed with smells, tastes, and flavors!

Andrew is a pioneer in the food and beverage landscape and is currently working with celebrity chefs to create infused dining events. He is one of the first people in the world to gain accreditation from the American Culinary Federation with a certificate in "Cannabis Cuisine and Edibles." Andrew is also one of just a few Canadian Wine Scholars as well as the holder of Level Three accreditation from WSET (the Wine & Spirit Education Trust).

Andrew's heavily researched opinions are very well received in his work as a speaker and content creator. His authentic, candid approach makes him relatable and trustworthy. He has been interviewed and quoted internationally in publications like the *LA Times*, *The Globe and Mail*, *High Times*, and many more.

Andrew is the founder and CEO of The Cannabis Sommelier, a full suite events production company focusing on cannabis-centric events. He is also the president of TCSA Consulting, a consulting agency in the adult-use cannabis space.

Andrew lives in the foothills of the Canadian Rocky Mountains in Calgary, Alberta, Canada, with his wife Sarah and their dog Zeus.

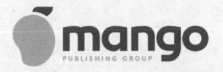

Mango Publishing, established in 2014, publishes an eclectic list of books by diverse authors—both new and established voices—on topics ranging from business, personal growth, women's empowerment, LGBTQ studies, health, and spirituality to history, popular culture, time management, decluttering, lifestyle, mental wellness, aging, and sustainable living. We were recently named 2019 *and* 2020's #1 fastest growing independent publisher by *Publishers Weekly.* Our success is driven by our main goal, which is to publish high quality books that will entertain readers as well as make a positive difference in their lives.

Our readers are our most important resource; we value your input, suggestions, and ideas. We'd love to hear from you— after all, we are publishing books for you!

Please stay in touch with us and follow us at:

Facebook: Mango Publishing

Twitter: @MangoPublishing

Instagram: @MangoPublishing

LinkedIn: Mango Publishing

Pinterest: Mango Publishing

Newsletter: mangopublishinggroup.com/newsletter

Join us on Mango's journey to reinvent publishing, one book at a time.

CPSIA information can be obtained
at www.ICGtesting.com
Printed in the USA
JSHW032004290523
42355JS00005B/5

9 781642 505528